Suggested citation:
> Haverkamp D, Espey D, Paisano R, Cobb N. Cancer Mortality Among American Indians and Alaska Natives: Regional Differences, 1999–2003. Indian Health Service. Rockville, MD, February 2008.

Available in Portable Document Format at:
> http://www.ihs.gov/medicalprograms/epi/index.cfm?
> module=health_issues&option=cancer&cat=sub_4

Note:
> The findings and conclusions in this report are those of the author(s) and do not necessarily represent the views of the Centers for Disease Control and Prevention or the Indian Health Service.

Cancer Mortality Among American Indians and Alaska Natives: Regional Differences, 1999–2003

Donald Haverkamp, MPH*
David Espey, MD*
Roberta Paisano, MHSA[†]
Nathaniel Cobb, MD[†]

February, 2008

*   Division of Cancer Prevention and Control, National Center for Chronic Disease Prevention and Health Promotion, Centers for Disease Control and Prevention, assigned to the Indian Health Service, Division of Epidemiology and Disease Prevention.

[†]   Division of Epidemiology and Disease Prevention, Office of Public Health Support, Indian Health Service.

CONTENTS   PAGE

Purpose and Description of Cancer Mortality Among American Indians and Alaska Natives: Regional Differences, 1999–2003

This monograph reports regional cancer mortality rates among American Indians and Alaska Natives (AI/ANs) within areas served by the U.S. Department of Health and Human Services (DHHS), Indian Health Service (IHS). These areas are comprised of certain counties found within 35 states. AI/ANs residing in these counties represent about 56% of the total AI/AN bridged single-race population in the United States. We present the cancer mortality rates for 1999–2003 for the principal cancer types and compare them with the general U.S. population rates during the same period. We also present the estimated IHS service population for each region. The purpose of this publication is to provide detailed information on the impact of cancer among AI/ANs, with a focus on the regional variability of cancer mortality for this population.

This publication was made possible by the partnership between the IHS Division of Epidemiology and Disease Prevention and the Centers for Disease Control and Prevention (CDC) Division of Cancer Prevention and Control, utilizing resources available from the National Cancer Institute, National Institutes of Health, and CDC's National Center for Health Statistics.

Overview of the Indian Health Service

IHS is responsible for providing health services to members of federally recognized AI/AN tribes on the basis of laws passed by the U.S. Congress pursuant to its authority to regulate commerce with the Indian nations as explicitly specified in the *U.S. Constitution* and in other pertinent authorities. On August 5, 1954, the Indian health program became a primary responsibility of the U.S. Public Health Service (USPHS) under the Transfer Act (Public Law 83-568). This act provides that all functions, responsibilities, authorities, and duties relating to the maintenance and operation of the hospital and health facilities for AI/ANs and the conservation of Indian health shall be administered by the Surgeon General of USPHS.[1]

The IHS mission, in partnership with AI/AN people, is to raise their physical, mental, social, and spiritual health to the highest level possible. The IHS goal is to ensure that comprehensive, culturally acceptable personal and public health services are available and accessible to all AI/AN people. To carry out this goal, IHS acts as the principal federal health advocate for Indian people.[2]

IHS has implemented its responsibility by developing and operating a health service delivery system designed to provide a broad-spectrum program of preventive, curative, rehabilitative, and environmental services. This system integrates health services delivered directly through IHS facilities and staff with those purchased by IHS through contractual arrangements, taking into account other health resources to which AI/ANs have access. Tribes are also actively involved in program implementation.

Two key laws enacted to improve the health status of AI/ANs are described as follows:

- The 1975 Indian Self-Determination and Education Assistance Act, Public Law 93-638, as amended, builds on IHS programs in their communities and provides funding for improvement of tribal capability to contract under the act.[3] Under this act, tribes can chose to continue to receive health services provided directly by IHS or they can opt to take control of their own health-care services by managing IHS funding directly. They can also selectively manage certain components of their health services and leave others to IHS. Approximately half of the IHS budget is transferred directly to tribes under self-governance arrangements, and more tribes are expected to do so in the future. As these tribes move to self-governance for health services, they are going to rely increasingly on regional health profiles to guide them in strategic planning for optimal use of these resources.

- The 1976 Indian Health Care Improvement Act, Public Law 94-437, as amended, was intended to elevate the health status of AI/ANs to a level equal to that of the general population through a program of authorized higher resource levels in the IHS budget.[4] Appropriated resources were used to expand health services, build and renovate medical facilities, and set up the construction of safe drinking water and sanitary disposal facilities. It also established programs designed to increase the number of AI/AN health professionals and to improve health-care access for AI/AN people living in urban areas.

Indian Health Service Structure

The IHS health services delivery system is managed through local administrative units. A service unit is the basic health organization for a geographic area served by IHS, just as a county or city health department is the basic health organization in a state health department. These are defined areas, usually centered around a single federal reservation within the continental United States, or a population concentration in Alaska. A limited number of service units cover multiple small reservations; certain large reservations are divided into multiple service units. All of IHS service units are grouped into the following 12 larger cultural-demographic management jurisdictions known as IHS Area offices:[5]

Aberdeen	Billings	Oklahoma
Alaska	California	Phoenix
Albuquerque	Nashville	Portland
Bemidji	Navajo	Tucson

As of January 2007, the Area offices consisted of 164 IHS and tribally managed service units. IHS operated 33 hospitals, 52 health centers, 38 health stations, and two school health centers. AI tribes and AN corporations operated 15 hospitals, 220 health centers, 116 health stations, 162 Alaska village clinics, and nine school health centers.[6]

Cancer Mortality Among AI/ANs: Regional Differences, 1999–2003

INTRODUCTION

IHS has strived to improve the health of AI/ANs in the United States for >50 years. The results have been marked decreases in infectious disease mortality and infant and maternal mortality. Since 1973, life expectancy at birth for AI/ANs nationally has increased by >9 years and is now at 74.5 years. However, this is still approximately 2.4 years less than that for the U.S. general population.[7] With these improvements in health status and increased life span, chronic diseases have begun to impact heavily on the AI/AN community. Malignant neoplasms are the second leading cause of death for AI/ANs throughout the country.[8] In Alaska, cancer is the leading cause of death among ANs.[9] Although the majority of detailed cancer surveillance, including cancer mortality, has focused on AI/AN populations in the Southwest and Alaska [10-18], selected authors have examined cancer trends nationally.[19-23]

In 1997, Cobb and Paisano examined cancer mortality trends for 1989–1993 for AI/AN populations residing in counties on or near Indian reservations.[24] They reported that the AI/AN population had overall lower cancer mortality when examined nationally, yet displayed marked regional variation when examined at the IHS Area level. Garguillo et al. reported trends in mortality for four major cancers (lung/bronchus, colorectal, prostate, and breast) by sex and race/ethnicity for 1990–1998. They determined that cancer mortality among AI/AN either increased for a given cancer and sex while decreasing in other major racial/ethnic groups (most common), or AI/AN experienced proportionally greater increases or proportionally smaller decreases in cancer mortality (prostate).[22] Because they did not attempt to adjust for the known racial misclassification for AI/ANs in state vital records, the rates are probably underestimates. Consequently, the disparities would likely be greater if racial misclassification were accounted for.[25, 26] Espey et al. compared 1990–1995 with 1996–2001 data and determined that there was an increase in cancer mortality during the latter period for AI/ANs, whereas cancer mortality had decreased in the United States for all races combined.[21]

Initial IHS cancer mortality monographs [24, 27] reported cancer mortality data for the 12 IHS administrative Areas (IHS Areas).[5] The tables and charts in the most recent IHS cancer mortality monograph depicted broader geographic regions instead of IHS Areas.[20] In this monograph, mortality rates are again reported by geographic region, with the addition of a sixth region (Southern Plains).

These studies and publications revealed certain key points. First, U.S. AI/AN mortality rates differ substantially from U.S. rates for all races combined. Second, marked regional differences exist in rates of cancer mortality and incidence among AI/ANs in the United States. Third, recent trends in AI/AN cancer mortality are substantially different and typically less favorable, compared with other major racial/ethnic groups. Most of these studies used different methodologies and different study periods, making comparisons difficult. This report provides data regarding cancer mortality among AI/ANs and, by using similar methods, allows comparison with data collected during previous periods.

METHODS AND SOURCES OF DATA

Denominators — IHS Service Population and United States All-races Population
All mortality rates and population estimates for this monograph were calculated using SEER*Stat (Surveillance Epidemiology and End Results), Version 6.3.5 (available at http://seer.cancer.gov/seerstat/).[28] CDC's National Center for Health Statistics (NCHS) provides the underlying mortality data for SEER*Stat databases. The IHS service population counts used in this monograph are based on U.S. Census Bureau intercensal county population estimates, updated in February 2006, after adjustments based on the 2000 census were made under an interagency agreement between the National Institutes of Health (NIH)/National Cancer Institute (NCI) and the U.S. Census Bureau. During the decennial census, the U.S. Census Bureau enumerates those persons who identify themselves as AI/AN. The intercensal estimates are developed by using a co-hort-component method whereby each component of population change — births, deaths, domestic migration, and international migration — is estimated separately for each birth cohort by sex, race, and Hispanic origin.[29] The IHS service population is es-timated by including only AI/ANs who reside in counties in which IHS has clinical facili-ties or that are in or adjacent to federally recognized Indian lands (IHS service areas). These counties are referred to by IHS as contract health service delivery areas (CHSDA). The IHS service population refers to the AI/AN population residing in CHSDA counties — regardless if they use IHS services.

County-level population estimates from the U.S. Census Bureau that were modified by NCI were used as denominators in the rate calculations.[30] The 2000 census allowed respondents to identify themselves as multiracial. Because of this, NCHS and the U.S. Census Bureau developed bridging methods for single-race estimates to describe long-term trends in disease.[31] This bridging method has a substantial impact on AI/AN bridged population counts. For the United States as a whole, the bridged AI/AN popu-lation count is 12.0% higher than the single-race count.

During 1999–2003, the average annual IHS service population was 1,694,439 per-sons, whereas the average for the entire AI/AN bridged single-race population in the United States was estimated at 3,007,510 persons (Table 1, columns 2 and 3). Of the six regions chosen for this monograph, the Southwest region has the largest IHS ser-vice population (approximately 520,437 persons), distributed in five states and includ-ing four IHS Areas (Figure 1). Next is the Pacific Coast region (369,217 persons), rep-resenting five states and two IHS Areas. The Southern Plains region, representing three states and two IHS Areas, has 327,262 persons. The Northern Plains region, representing 11 states and three IHS Areas, has 265,912 persons. Alaska (108,462 persons) represents one state and one IHS Area, and the East region, representing 25 states and Washington, DC, and one IHS Area, has 103,149 persons. This distribution is represented in Table 1. Of note is that the population included in these regions does not reflect the concentration of AI/ANs in the United States. Rather, it is becoming a standard method for analyzing and presenting AI/AN-specific data (see Change to Regional Analyses on page 7 of this monograph). There are several precedents for using regional analyses when analyzing AI/AN populations data.[19-23, 32, 33]

To remain consistent with past versions of the monograph, the United States all-race population rate was used as a reference group for comparison to the regional AI/AN rates. This reference group included all race/ethnic groups, including AI/AN, and included all fifty states and Washington, D.C. Although not presented in this report, the authors also compared regional AI/AN rates to rates among Non-Hispanic whites. Tables showing these comparisons can be found at the IHS Division of Epidemiology and Disease Prevention website (http://www.ihs.gov/medicalprograms/epi/index.cfm?module=health_issues&option=cancer&cat=sub_4). Not all states in the United States contain IHS service areas. In the 35 states that do, only a subset of counties are service/CHSDA counties. Figure 1 displays the states and CHSDA counties within each of the six regions used in this analysis. On the basis of the intercensal population estimates, approximately 56% of all AI/ANs in the United States reside within the geographic boundaries of the IHS service areas.

Figure 1. CHSDA Counties Used in Cancer Mortality Analyses for the AI/AN Population by Region

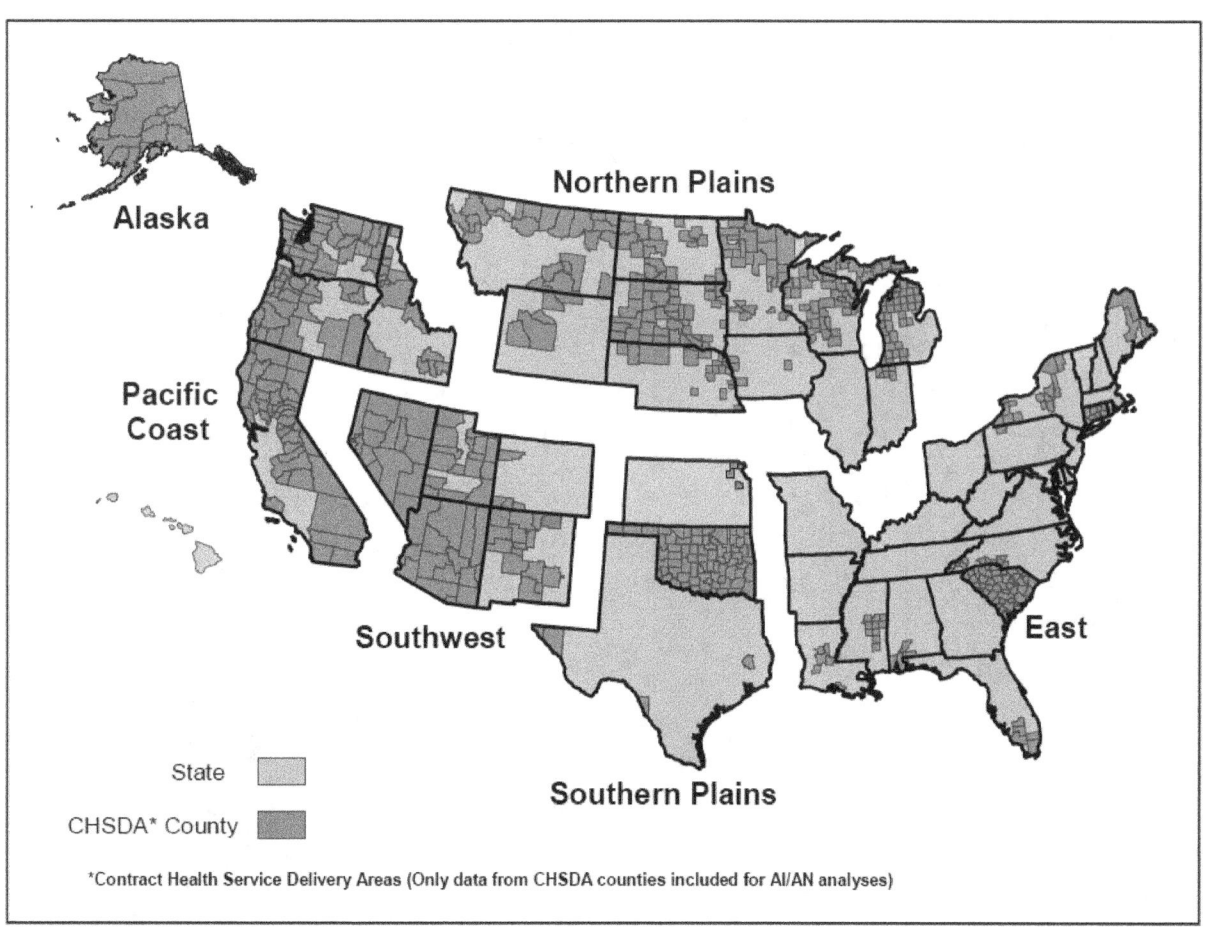

*Contract Health Service Delivery Areas (Only data from CHSDA counties included for AI/AN analyses)

Numerator — Mortality Data

AI/AN vital event statistics are derived from data furnished by NCHS, who obtains birth and death records for all U.S. residents from the state health departments, on the basis of information reported on official state birth and death certificates. The records received from NCHS by IHS do not contain names, addresses, tribal identity, or medical record identification numbers. Each record includes the single underlying cause of death and is determined according to standard criteria and data listed on the death certificate. The records also contain county of residence, which allows selection of deaths of residents in counties located within IHS service areas. These investigators examined only those AI/AN deaths for 1999–2003 in which the underlying cause of death was cancer, as determined by *International Classification of Diseases, 10th Revision* (ICD-10) codes in the range of C00–C97 (Table 2).

The AI/AN vital events data in this publication pertain only to those AI/ANs residing at the time of their death in the counties that constitute the IHS service areas. By limiting the analysis to the AI/AN populations of IHS service counties where more awareness of AI/AN racial/ethnic identity exists, racial misclassification is minimized.[34]

Because the AI/AN population is considerably younger than the U.S. all races population (Figures 2 and 3), and for reasons of comparability with recent analyses and publications, mortality rates presented in this report have been age-adjusted by the direct method, using the 2000 U.S. population as the age standard. An adjusted rate that was computed on the basis of a limited number of deaths should be interpreted with caution, because the adjusted rate might differ from the underlying rate. Cell suppressions were not applied in the case of small numbers, due to the desire of AI/AN populations to present these data, which have typically been suppressed in the past.

Figure 2

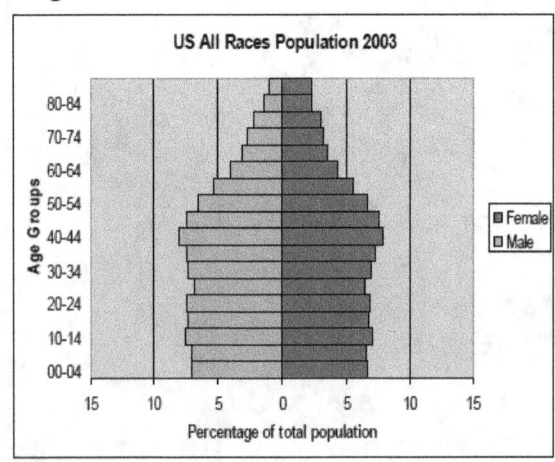

Figure 3

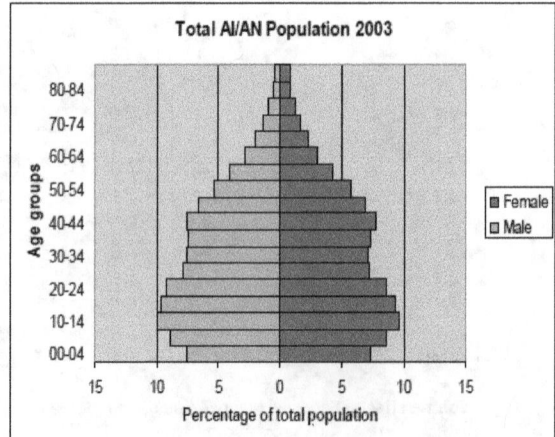

Change to Regional Analyses

The first two monographs presenting cancer mortality data for AI/AN used the IHS areas as the geographic unit of analysis.[24, 27] Although convenient and of interest for programmatic purposes, this approach posed problems. First, certain area rates were not stable because of a relatively limited number of cases. Second, certain counties were split between two or more IHS Areas; therefore, cases were arbitrarily assigned to one IHS Area or the other on the basis of their percentage coverage of that county. Lastly, use of IHS Area boundaries could imply tribal affiliation, to which tribal leaders and members might object. Despite the breakout of rates by IHS Area, the distinct patterns were often more regionally specific than IHS Area-specific. On the basis of these considerations, the ensuing monograph used broader regions of the country as the geographic unit of analysis, as opposed to IHS administrative areas. As in the previous reports, the analysis was restricted to CHSDA/service counties to mitigate the effects of misclassification. Since then an additional region has been proposed and this monograph includes this new region in calculating cancer mortality rates among AI/ANs. The new "Southern Plains" region was proposed as a result of feedback from several tribes in both eastern and southern plains states, stating that the cancer mortality rates of the original "East" region were not representative of the rates that they saw among their own populations. This regional approach addresses certain limitations of the IHS Area analysis and offers more stable rates on which to base programmatic decisions. It also offers a more standard approach by using state and county boundaries that are more consistent with census data and with analyses used by other entities. An additional method used to control for fluctuation in rates that occur when a relatively limited population and number of deaths exist is the aggregation of data throughout a 5-year period.

Analysis

Data were examined for all cancer deaths combined as well as for leading cancer sites and sites. Average annual age-adjusted mortality rates were calculated by using the estimated 1999–2003 population for each Region (Table 1, column 2). To compute 95% confidence intervals (CIs) for each rate, we used the method described by Fay and Feuer.[35] We also calculated mortality rate ratios (MRRs) and 95% CIs, using the Breslow and Day method, to compare the relative difference in age-adjusted mortality rates with the U.S. general (USG) population for the same period.[36]

RESULTS

During 1999–2003, the average annual age-adjusted cancer mortality rate among AI/AN for all cancers for both sexes combined was 161.9/100,000 population for all regions combined. This rate was significantly lower than the rate for U.S. all races of 195.7/100,000 population (MRR, 0.83; CI, 0.81–0.85). Males had greater cancer mortality (191.2/100,000 population) than females (141.9/100,000 population), but both groups had significantly lower mortality when compared with the USG population (MRR, 0.78; CI 0.76–0.81 for males and MRR, 0.86; CI 0.84–0.89 for females).

Marked variation occurred among regions; the Southwest, East, Pacific Coast, and Southern Plains all had rates below the USG population (MRRs, 0.67, 0.71, 0.72 and 0.79, respectively). Alaska and the Northern Plains had higher rates (MRR, 1.24 and 1.30, respectively) for all cancers, both sexes combined. For all regions combined, MRRs for 12 leading causes of cancer death are illustrated in Figures 4–6. Tables of MMRs for specific cancer sites (by sex and region) are accessible at the IHS Division of Epidemiology and Disease Prevention website (http://www.ihs.gov/ medicalprograms/epi/index.cfm?module=health_issues&option=cancer&cat=sub_4).

Lung cancer was the leading cause of cancer mortality in the United States as well as for the IHS service population overall (Table 16). Among AI/AN populations, for all regions combined, lung cancer was followed by colorectal cancer, miscellaneous malignant cancer, and breast and prostate cancers. Lung cancer was the leading cause of cancer death in all regions except the Southwest, where the leading category of cancer death for female and both sexes combined was miscellaneous malignant cancer. When we examined cancer mortality rates by specific cancer site and by sex, substantial variations among the regions were evident. Detailed results for 12 cancer sites are displayed in Figures 7–37 and Tables 3–15. For each region, the five leading causes of cancer mortality are listed in Table 16.

DISCUSSION

The data presented here demonstrate that the cancer mortality burden among AI/ANs throughout the United States is different from that of the USG population. In general, AI/ANs in the Southwest, East, Southern Plains, and Pacific Coast regions had lower cancer mortality rates than those in the northern part of the country. However, within any geographic region, mortality rates for specific cancers were not all lower or higher than the U.S. rates. For each specific type of cancer and for each sex, varying rankings by region were identified.

The variability in lung and bronchus cancer mortality observed among AI/ANs across regions (highest in Northern Plains, lowest in Southwest) is likely a consequence of the variability in tobacco use. Smoking prevalence among AI/AN adults is approximately 20% in the Southwest but is approximately 44% in both the northern plains and Alaska regions.[23] Regional variability in cancer mortality for other cancers is more difficult to explain and might be linked to differences in diet, prevalence of obesity and alcoholism, or access to care or later stage diagnoses.

Limitations are well-recognized in using death certificate data to examine cause-specific mortality. These include racial misclassification, errors in listing the decedent's residence at time of death, and errors in reporting the precise cause of death. Studies have reported that racial misclassification of AI/ANs on death certificates is a problem in certain regions of the country.[25, 26, 37] Additionally, data indicate that AI/ANs die more often than whites of what is termed "signs, symptoms, and ill-defined conditions".[38] These two latter problems lead to underestimations of the overall cancer mortality rates as well as underestimations of mortality for specific types of cancer. Our analysis provides evidence that miscellaneous malignant cancers are the leading cause of cancer mortality among the AI/AN population of the Southwest (for females and both sexes combined).

An additional limitation is that certain rates published in this monograph are based on only a limited number of cases. These have been included because AI/AN communities have expressed the need to no longer suppress these data; however, such rates should be interpreted with caution. The results of tests of statistical significance are noted for all comparisons with U.S. all-race rates in Tables 3–15.

All rates in this report were age-adjusted using the 2000 U.S. standard population to make them more comparable with current publications. Rates from previous IHS cancer mortality reports were based on the 1970 U.S. standard population. Changing to the 2000 U.S. standard population affects the magnitude of the rates. Cancer mortality rates based on the 2000 U.S. population may be higher than those calculated using the U.S. 1970 population since the 2000 U.S. population has an older age distribution, and cancer is more prevalent in older persons.

Although we used recently published census estimates, the degree to which errors might have occurred in the accurate counting of AI/ANs is not known precisely. However, evidence indicates that any errors would likely result in undercounting. Errors in using population figures that might be lower than the true numbers might lead to over-estimation of the true cancer mortality rates for regions of the country where this was a problem.

Despite these limitations and changes, the findings included here clearly demonstrate that AI/ANs across the country experience different cancer mortality patterns both between regions and in comparison with U.S. all-race rates, and that AI/ANs in the Southwest have markedly different cancer mortality patterns from other AI/ANs in the United States.

To better understand the extent of cancer mortality among AI/ANs in the United States, further collaboration between CDC, IHS, and state vital records offices should be promoted and expanded. A study is underway that links IHS patient registration data with vital records data from approximately 25 states to identify AI/AN persons who have been misclassified as non-Native. Such collaborations can provide improved data for developing preventive programs and intervention strategies that should be targeted appropriately for specific populations. Improved cancer mortality data can illuminate the extent of the problem and help provide direction to decision makers regarding where to apply limited resources for the most beneficial impact.

REFERENCES

1. Grim C. IHS Marks 50 Years Providing Service. *US Medicine.* January 2006.

2. Indian Health Service Fact Sheet http://info.ihs.gov/Files/IHSFacts-Jan2007.doc. Accessed June 15, 2007.

3. PL (Public Law) 93 – 638. http://www.ihs.gov/NonMedicalPrograms/chr/pl93-638.cfm. Accessed June 15, 2007.

4. Indian Health Care Improvement Act http://info.ihs.gov/TreatiesLaws/Treaties3.pdf. Accessed January 14, 2007.

5. Indian Health Service: Area Offices and Facilities. http://www.ihs.gov/FacilitiesServices/AreaOffices/AreaOffices_index.asp. Accessed May 20, 2007.

6. Indian Health Service: Year 2007 Profile. http://info.ihs.gov/Files/ProfileSheet-Jan2007.doc. Accessed January 14, 2007.

7. Indian Health Service: A Quick Look http://info.ihs.gov/Files/QuickLook-Jan2007.doc. Accessed June 14, 2007.

8. Indian Health Service: Trends in Indian Health, 1998-1999. Rockville, MD; 2000.

9. Lanier AP, Kelly JJ, Maxwell J, McEvoy T, Homan C. Cancer in Alaska Native people, 1969-2003. *Alaska Med.* Jul-Sep 2006;48(2):30-59.

10. Brown MO, Lanier AP, Becker TM. Colorectal cancer incidence and survival among Alaska Natives, 1969-1993. *Int J Epidemiol.* Jun 1998;27(3):388-396.

11. Chao A, Becker TM, Jordan SW, Darling R, Gilliland FD, Key CR. Decreasing rates of cervical cancer among American Indians and Hispanics in New Mexico (United States). *Cancer Causes Control.* Mar 1996;7(2):205-213.

12. Chao A, Gilliland FD, Hunt WC, Bulterys M, Becker TM, Key CR. Increasing incidence of colon and rectal cancer among Hispanics and American Indians in New Mexico (United States), 1969-94. *Cancer Causes Control.* Mar 1998;9(2):137-144.

13. Eidson M, Becker TM, Wiggins CL, Key CR, Samet JM. Breast cancer among Hispanics, American Indians and non-Hispanic whites in New Mexico. *Int J Epidemiol.* Apr 1994;23(2):231-237.

14. Lanier AP, Kelly JJ, Holck P, Smith B, McEvoy T, Sandidge J. Cancer incidence in Alaska Natives thirty-year report 1969-1998. *Alaska Med.* Oct-Dec 2001;43(4):87-115.

15. Lanier AP, Kelly JJ, Smith B, et al. Alaska Native cancer update: incidence rates 1989-1993. *Cancer Epidemiol Biomarkers Prev.* Sep 1996;5(9):749-751.

16. Schiff M, Becker TM, Smith HO, Gilliland FD, Key CR. Ovarian cancer incidence and mortality in American Indian, Hispanic, and non-Hispanic white women in New Mexico. *Cancer Epidemiol Biomarkers Prev.* May 1996;5(5):323-327.

17. Schiff M, Key CR, Gilliland FD, Becker TM. Ethnic differences in uterine corpus cancer incidence and mortality in New Mexico's American Indians, hispanics and non-Hispanic whites. *Int J Epidemiol.* Apr 1997;26(2):249-255.

18. Wiggins CL, Becker TM, Key CR, Samet JM. Stomach cancer among New Mexico's American Indians, Hispanic whites, and non-Hispanic whites. *Cancer Res.* Mar 15 1989;49(6):1595-1599.

19. Cobb N, Paisano RE. Patterns of cancer mortality among Native Americans. *Cancer.* Dec 1 1998;83(11):2377-2383.

20. Espey D, Paisano RE, and Cobb N. Cancer Mortality among American Indians and Alaska Natives: Regional Differences, 1994-1998. Rockville, MD: Indian Health Service; 2003.

21. Espey D, Paisano R, Cobb N. Regional patterns and trends in cancer mortality among American Indians and Alaska Natives, 1990-2001. *Cancer.* Mar 1 2005;103(5):1045-1053.

22. Garguillo P, Wingo P, Coates R, Thompson T. Recent trends in mortality rates for four major cancers, by sex and race/ethnicity--United States, 1990-1998. *MMWR Morb Mortal Wkly Rep.* Jan 25 2002;51(3):49-53.

23. Espey DK, Wu XC, Swan J, et al. Annual report to the nation on the status of cancer, 1975-2004, featuring cancer in American Indians and Alaska Natives. *Cancer.* Oct 15 2007:2119-2152.

24. Cobb N PR. Cancer Mortality among American Indians and Alaska Natives in the United States: Regional Differences in Indian Health, 1989-1993. Indian Health Service: Rockville, MD; 1997.

25. Frost F, Shy KK. Racial differences between linked birth and infant death records in Washington State. *Am J Public Health.* Sep 1980;70(9):974-976.

26. Harwell TS, Hansen D, Moore KR, Jeanotte D, Gohdes D, Helgerson SD. Accuracy of race coding on American Indian death certificates, Montana 1996-1998. *Public Health Rep.* Jan-Feb 2002;117(1):44-49.

27. Valway S Kileen M, Paisano RE, Ortiz E. Cancer mortality among Native Americans in the United States: Regional Differences in Indian Health, 1984-1988 & Trends Over Time, 1968-1987. Indian Health Service: Rockville, MD; 1992.

28. Surveillance, Epidemiology, and End Results (SEER) Program (www.seer.cancer.gov) SEER*Stat Database: Mortality - All COD, Public-Use With County, Total U.S. (1990-2003) - Linked To County Attributes - Total U.S., 1969-2003 Counties, National Cancer Institute, DCCPS, Surveillance Research Program, Cancer Statistics Branch, released April 2006. Underlying mortality data provided by NCHS (www.cdc.gov/nchs).

29. 1990-2003, Expanded Races: (White, Black, American Indian/Alaska Native, Asian/Pacific Islander) by Origin (Hispanic, Non-Hispanic). http://seer.cancer.gov/popdata/download.html. Accessed Dec 11, 2006.

30. Surveillance, Epidemiology, and End Results (SEER) Program. Statistical Resources. U.S. population data 1969-2004. http://seer.cancer.gov/resources. Accessed July 9, 2007.

31. U.S. census populations with bridged race categories. http://www.cdc.gov/nchs/about/major/dvs/popbridge/popbridge.htm. Accessed July 9, 2007.

32. Denny CH, Holtzman D, Cobb N. Surveillance for health behaviors of American Indians and Alaska Natives. Findings from the Behavioral Risk Factor Surveillance System, 1997-2000. *MMWR Surveill Summ.* Aug 1 2003;52(7):1-13.

33. Wong D SE, Paisano EL, Cheek JE Indian Health Surveillance Report— Sexually Transmitted Diseases 2004. Atlanta, GA: U.S. Department of Health and Human Services, Centers for Disease Control and Prevention and Indian Health Service; 2006.

34. *Adjusting for Miscoding of Indian Race on State Death Certificates.* Rockville, MD: Division of Program Statistics, Indian Health Service; 1997.

35. Fay MP, Feuer EJ. Confidence intervals for directly standardized rates: a method based on the gamma distribution. *Stat Med.* Apr 15 1997;16(7):791-801.

36. Breslow NE, Day N. *Statistical methods in cancer research. Volume II - the design and analysis of cohort studies*: Oxford University Press; 1991.

37. Percy C, Stanek E, 3rd, Gloeckler L. Accuracy of cancer death certificates and its effect on cancer mortality statistics. *Am J Public Health.* Mar 1981;71(3):242-250.

38. Becker TM, Wiggins CL, Key CR, Samet JM. Symptoms, signs, and ill-defined conditions: a leading cause of death among minorities. *Am J Epidemiol.* Apr 1990;131(4):664-668.

Table 1. Definition of geographic regions, corresponding IHS service populations, total AI/AN population of states included in regions, and service population percentage — 1999–2003

Geographic region	IHS service population estimates*	Total AI/AN population estimates [†]	Service population % of total AI/AN	States (IHS administrative areas) [§]
Alaska	108,462	108,462	100%	**AK** (Alaska)
East	103,149	682,523	15.1 %	**AL**, AR, **CT**, DE, **FL**, GA, KY, **LA, ME**, MD, **MA, MS**, MO, NH, NJ, **NY, NC**, OH, **PA, RI, SC**, TN, VT, VA, WV, DC (Nashville)
Northern Plains	265,912	451,769	58.9 %	IL, **IN, IA, MI, MN, MT, NE, ND, SD, WI, WY** (Aberdeen, Bemidji, Billings)
Pacific Coast	369,217	669,090	55.2 %	**CA, ID, OR, WA**, HI (California, Portland)
Southern Plains	327,262	498,368	65.7 %	**KS, OK, TX** (Nashville, Oklahoma)
Southwest	520,437	597,299	87.1 %	**AZ, CO, NV, NM, UT** (Albuquerque, Navajo, Phoenix, Tucson)
All regions combined	1,694,439	3,007,510	56.3 %	

*All population figures are derived from intercensal estimates and annualized for 1999–2003 (updated February 2006).
[†] This total is derived from bridged single-race estimates.
[§] Bolded states contain CHSDA counties.

Table 2. Cancer site groupings for ICD-10–coded mortality data

Cancer-related causes of death	ICD-10
All malignant cancers	C00-C97
Oral cavity and pharynx	
Lip	C00
Tongue	C01–C02
Salivary gland	C07–C08
Floor of mouth	C04
Gum and other mouth	C03, C05–C06
Nasopharynx	C11
Tonsil	C09
Oropharynx	C10
Hypopharynx	C12–C13
Other oral cavity and pharynx	C14
Digestive system	
Esophagus	C15
Stomach	C16
Small intestine	C17
Colon and rectum	
Colon excluding rectum	C18, C26.0
Rectum and rectosigmoid junction	C19–C20
Anus, anal canal and anorectum	C21
Liver and intrahepatic bile duct	
Liver	C22.0, C22.2–C22.4, C22.7, C22.9
Intrahepatic bile duct	C22.1
Gallbladder	C23
Other biliary	C24
Pancreas	C25
Retroperitoneum	C48.0
Peritoneum, omentum, and mesentery	C45.1, C48.1–C48.2
Other digestive organs	C26.8–C26.9, C48.8

Table 2. Cancer site groupings for ICD-10–coded mortality data (continued)

Cancer-related causes of death	ICD-10
Respiratory system	
Nose, nasal cavity, and middle ear	C30–C31
Larynx	C32
Lung and bronchus	C34
Pleura	C38.4, C45.0
Trachea, mediastinum, and other respiratory organs	C33, C38.1–C38.3, C38.8, C39
Bones and joints	C40–C41
Soft tissue, including heart	C47, C49, C38.0, C45.2
Skin, excluding basal and squamous	
Melanoma of the Skin	C43
Other nonepithelial skin	C44, C46
Breast	C50
Female genital system	
Cervix uteri	C53
Corpus and uterus, NOS*	
Corpus uteri	C54
Uterus, NOS*	C55
Ovary	C56
Vagina	C52
Vulva	C51
Other female genital organs	C57–C58
Male genital system	
Prostate	C61
Testis	C62
Penis	C60
Other male genital organs	C63
Urinary system	
Urinary bladder	C67
Kidney and renal pelvis	C64–C65
Ureter	C66
Other urinary organs	C68
Eye and orbit	C69

Table 2. Cancer site groupings for ICD-10–coded mortality data (continued)

Cancer-related causes of death	ICD-10
Brain and other nervous system	C70, C71, C72
Endocrine system	
Thyroid	C73
Other endocrine including thymus	C37, C74–C75
Lymphoma	
Hodgkin lymphoma	C81
Non-Hodgkin lymphoma	C82–C85, C96.3
Myeloma	C90.0, C90.2
Leukemia	
Lymphocytic leukemia	
Acute lymphocytic leukemia	C91.0
Chronic lymphocytic leukemia	C91.1
Other lymphocytic leukemia	C91.2–C91.4, C91.7, C91.9
Myeloid and monocytic leukemia	
Acute myeloid	C92.0, C92.4–C92.5, C94.0, C94.2
Acute monocytic leukemia	C93.0
Chronic myeloid leukemia	C92.1
Other myeloid/monocytic leukemia	C92.2–C92.3, C92.7, C92.9, C93.1–C93.2, C93.7, C93.9
Other leukemia	
Other acute leukemia	C94.4, C94.5, C95.0
Aleukemic, subleukemic and NOS*	C90.1, C91.5, C94.1, C94.3, C94.7, C95.1, C95.2, C95.7, C95.9
Mesothelioma	C45
Kaposi Sarcoma	C46
Miscellaneous malignant cancer	C26.1, C45.7, C45.9, C76–C80, C88, C96.0–C96.2, C96.7, C96.9, C97

* NOS = not otherwise specified.

Figure 4

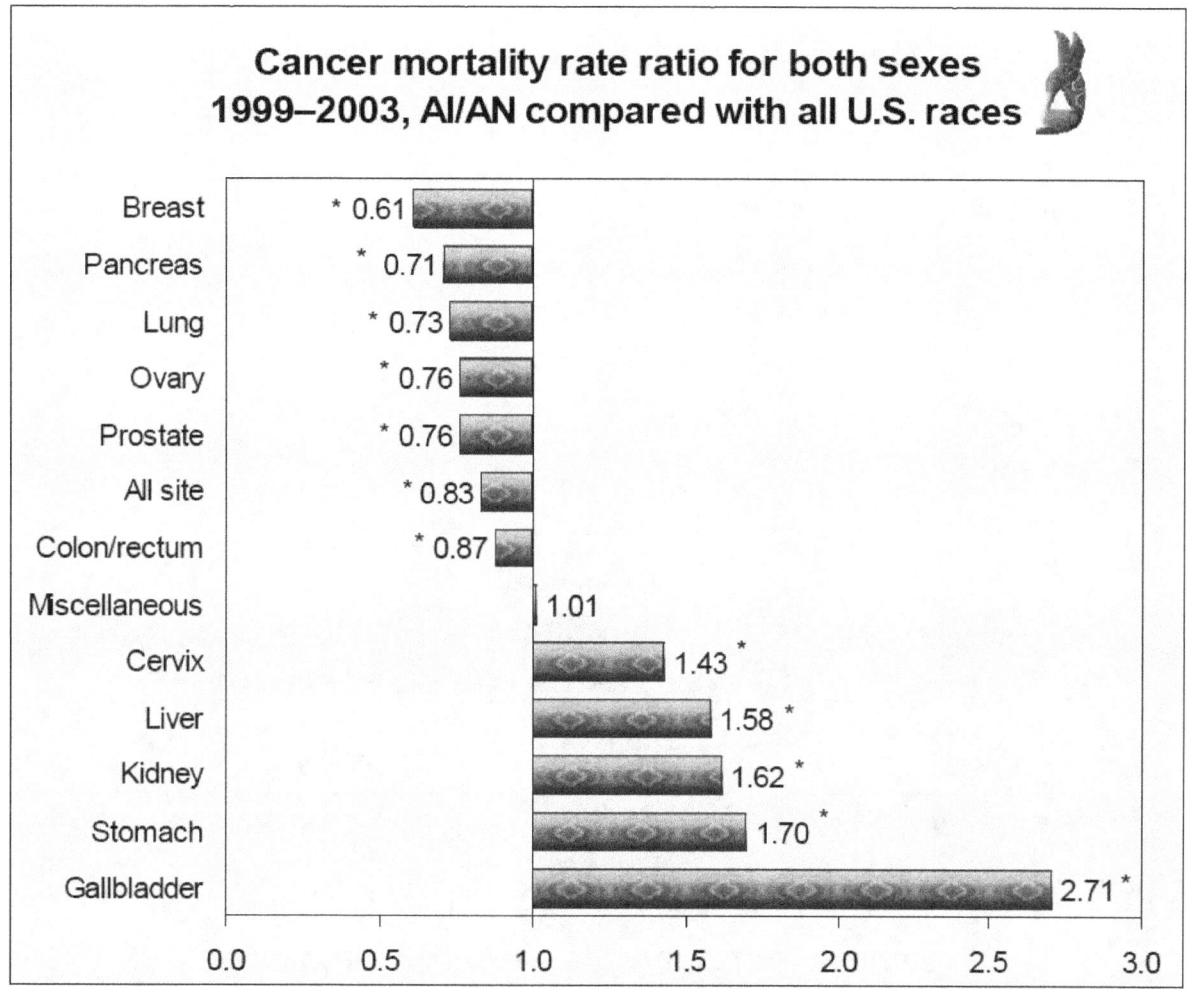

Cancer mortality rate ratio for both sexes 1999–2003, AI/AN compared with all U.S. races

Breast	* 0.61
Pancreas	* 0.71
Lung	* 0.73
Ovary	* 0.76
Prostate	* 0.76
All site	* 0.83
Colon/rectum	* 0.87
Miscellaneous	1.01
Cervix	1.43 *
Liver	1.58 *
Kidney	1.62 *
Stomach	1.70 *
Gallbladder	2.71 *

*AI/AN rate statistically different from U.S. all-race death rate.

Figure 5

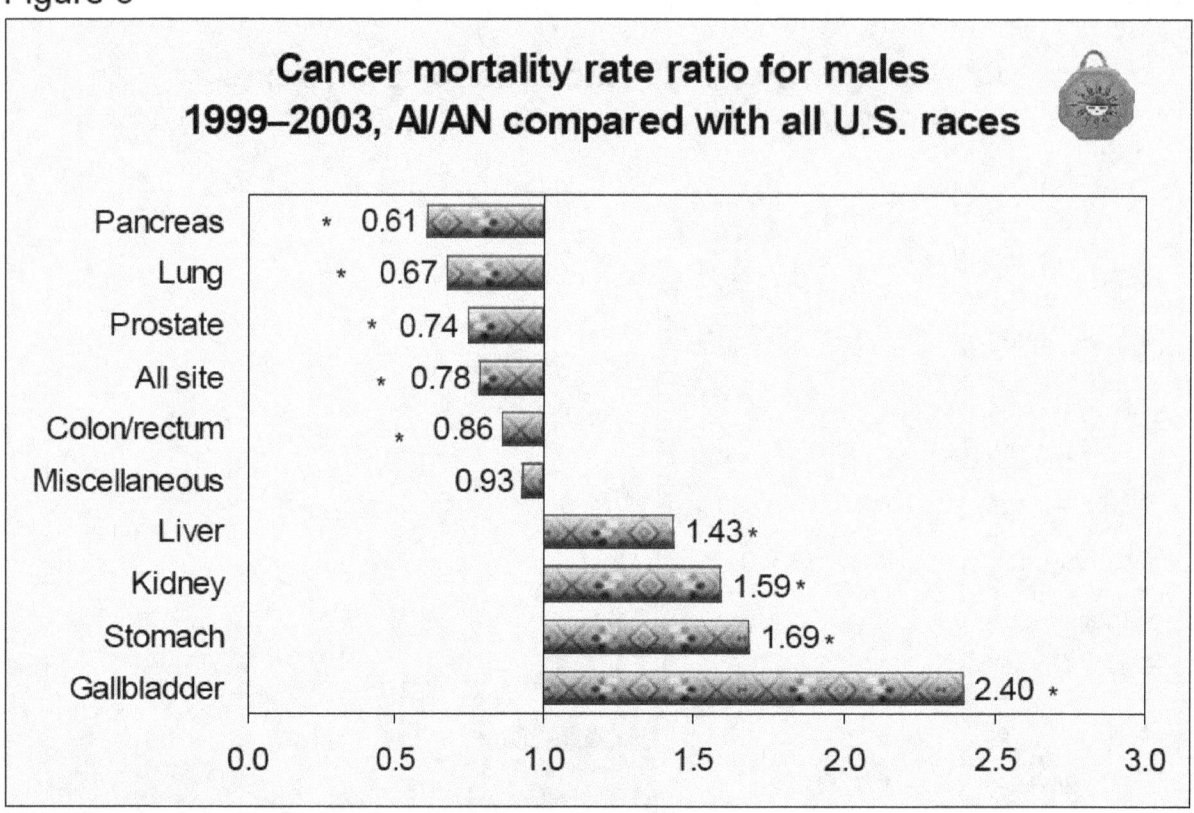

**Cancer mortality rate ratio for males
1999–2003, AI/AN compared with all U.S. races**

Pancreas	* 0.61
Lung	* 0.67
Prostate	* 0.74
All site	* 0.78
Colon/rectum	* 0.86
Miscellaneous	0.93
Liver	1.43 *
Kidney	1.59 *
Stomach	1.69 *
Gallbladder	2.40 *

0.0   0.5   1.0   1.5   2.0   2.5   3.0

*AI/AN rate statistically different from U.S. all-race death rate.

Figure 6

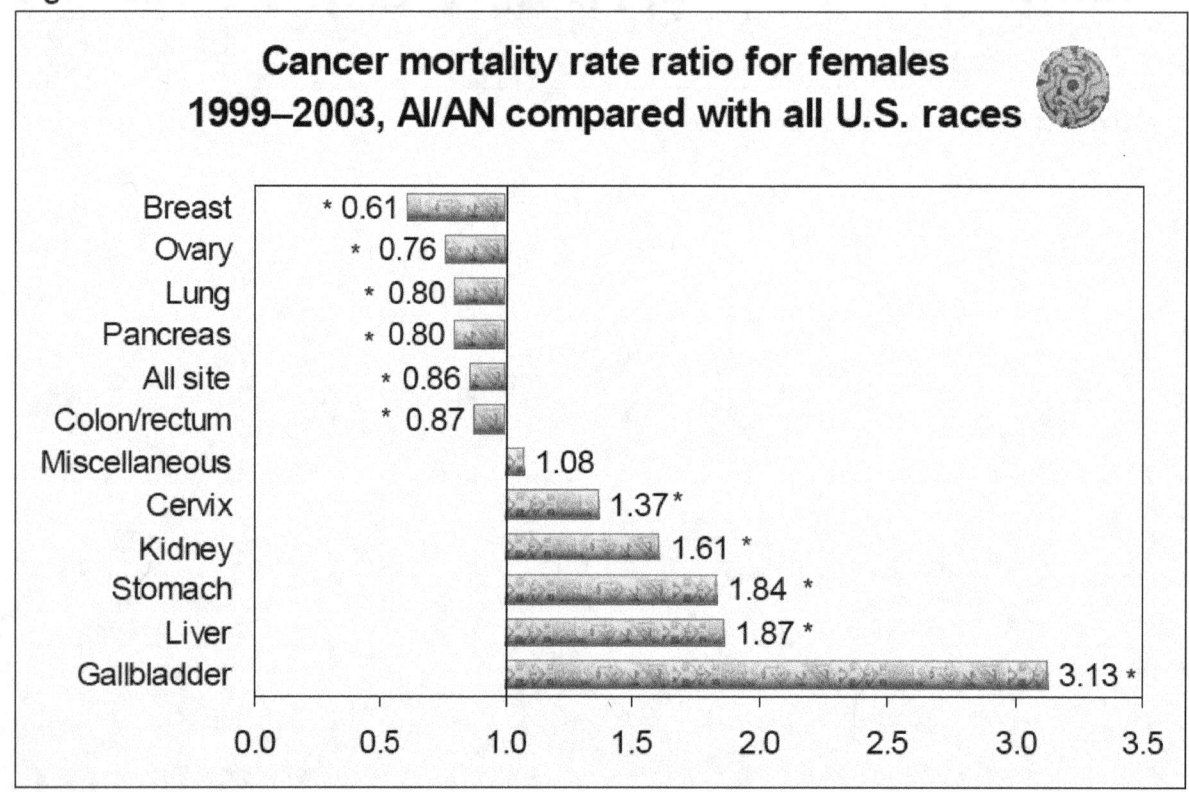

**Cancer mortality rate ratio for females
1999–2003, AI/AN compared with all U.S. races**

Breast	* 0.61
Ovary	* 0.76
Lung	* 0.80
Pancreas	* 0.80
All site	* 0.86
Colon/rectum	* 0.87
Miscellaneous	1.08
Cervix	1.37 *
Kidney	1.61 *
Stomach	1.84 *
Liver	1.87 *
Gallbladder	3.13 *

0.0   0.5   1.0   1.5   2.0   2.5   3.0   3.5

*AI/AN rate statistically different from U.S. all-race death rate.

Figure 7

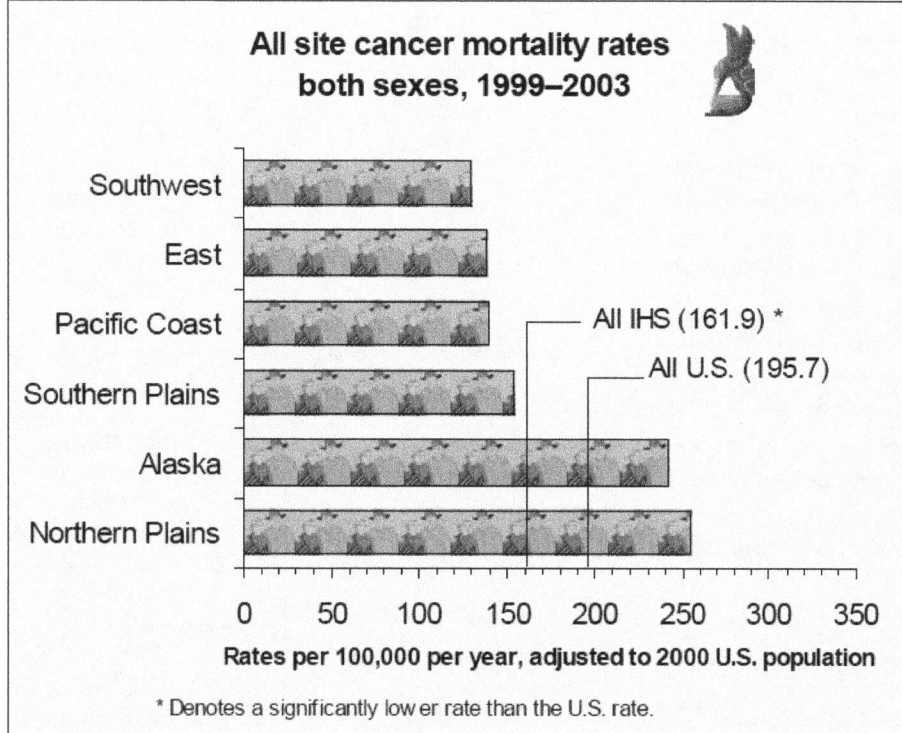

All site cancer mortality rates both sexes, 1999–2003

Southwest
East
Pacific Coast
Southern Plains
Alaska
Northern Plains

All IHS (161.9) *
All U.S. (195.7)

0   50   100   150   200   250   300   350

Rates per 100,000 per year, adjusted to 2000 U.S. population

* Denotes a significantly lower rate than the U.S. rate.

For both sexes combined, the 1999–2003 age-adjusted cancer mortality rate for all cancers combined is 161.9/100,000 among the entire IHS service population. This rate is significantly lower than the U.S. all-race combined rate for both sexes.

Regional rates demonstrate that both the Northern Plains and Alaska regions have significantly higher rates than the U.S. rate. The four remaining regions all have significantly lower rates than the U.S. rate for both sexes.

Table 3

Table 3 lists the total number of deaths caused by all cancers, 1999–2003, as well as mortality rates by IHS region for both sexes combined, males, and females.

Mortality rates are calculated per 100,000/ year and are age-adjusted to the 2000 U.S. population. Rates based on limited numbers of deaths should be interpreted with caution.

All site cancer mortality rates and total number of deaths, 1999–2003

	Both sexes		Males		Females	
	No.	Rate	No.	Rate	No.	Rate
U.S. all races	2,770,823	195.7	1,435,711	243.7	1,335,112	164.3
All IHS regions	7,227	161.9*	3,638	191.2*	3,589	141.9*
Alaska	660	242.3†	349	299.1†	311	205.4†
East	411	139.1*	203	155.0*	208	127.9*
Northern Plains	1,550	255.2†	774	305.5†	776	223.8†
Pacific Coast	1,303	140.2*	652	159.4*	651	126.7*
Southern Plains	1,586	154.5*	815	190.5*	771	131.2*
Southwest	1,717	130.2*	845	151.4*	872	115.5*

* Denotes a significantly lower rate than the U.S. rate.
† Denotes a significantly higher rate than the U.S. rate.

Figure 8

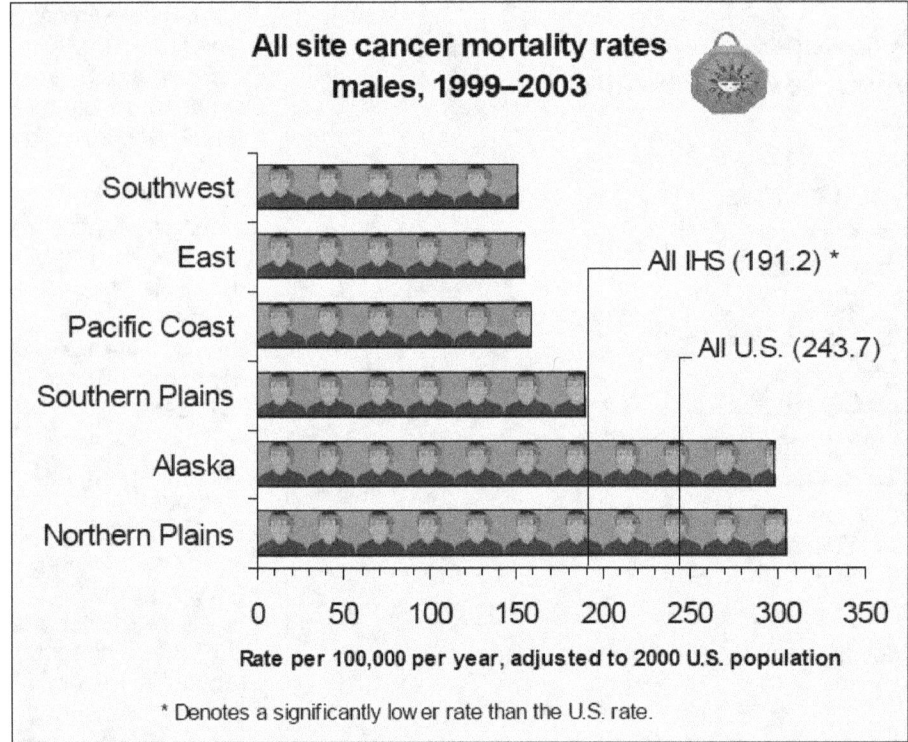

For males, the 1999–2003 age-adjusted cancer mortality rate for all cancers is 191.2/100,000 among the entire IHS service population. This rate is significantly lower than the U.S. all-race combined rate for males.

Regional rates reveal that both the Northern Plains and Alaska regions have significantly higher rates than the U.S. rate. The four remaining regions all have significantly lower rates than the U.S. rate for males.

Figure 9

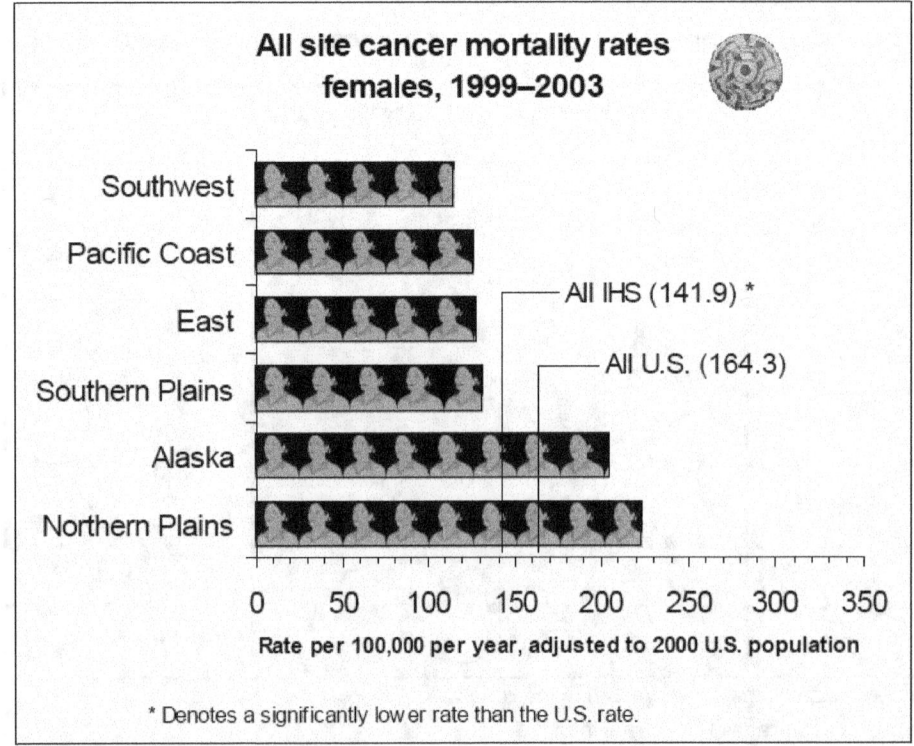

For females, the 1999–2003 age-adjusted cancer mortality rate for all cancers is 141.9/100,000 among the entire IHS service population. This rate is significantly lower than the U.S. all-race combined rate for females.

Regional rates reveal that both the Northern Plains and Alaska regions have significantly higher rates than the U.S. rate. The four remaining regions all have significantly lower rates than the U.S. rate for females.

Figure 10

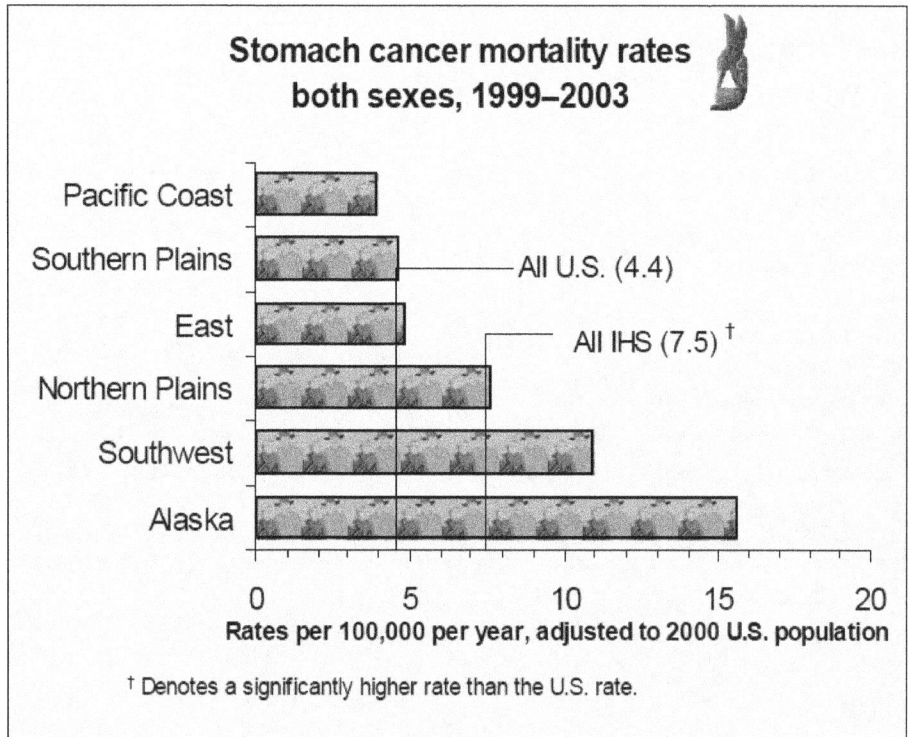

Stomach cancer mortality rates both sexes, 1999–2003

Pacific Coast
Southern Plains — All U.S. (4.4)
East — All IHS (7.5) [†]
Northern Plains
Southwest
Alaska

Rates per 100,000 per year, adjusted to 2000 U.S. population

[†] Denotes a significantly higher rate than the U.S. rate.

For both sexes combined, the 1999–2003 age-adjusted cancer mortality rate for stomach cancer is 7.5/100,000 among the entire IHS service population. This rate is significantly higher than the U.S. all-race combined rate for both sexes.

Regional rates reveal that the Alaska, Southwest, and Northern Plains regions have significantly higher rates than the U.S. rate for both sexes.

Table 4

Table 4 lists the total number of deaths caused by stomach cancer, 1999–2003, as well as mortality rates by IHS region for both sexes combined, males, and females.

Mortality rates are calculated per 100,000/year and are age-adjusted to the 2000 U.S. population. Rates based on limited numbers of deaths should be interpreted with caution.

Stomach cancer mortality rates and total number of deaths, 1999–2003						
	Both sexes		Males		Females	
	No.	Rate	No.	Rate	No.	Rate
U.S. all races	61,983	4.4	36,166	6.1	25,817	3.1
All IHS regions	329	7.5[†]	190	10.3[†]	139	5.7[†]
Alaska	46	15.7[†]	23	19.0[†]	23	14.0[†]
East	15	4.9	10	7.1	5	3.1
Northern Plains	48	7.7[†]	28	10.6[†]	20	5.9[†]
Pacific Coast	37	4.0	21	5.1	16	3.2
Southern Plains	48	4.7	28	6.7	20	3.5
Southwest	135	11.0[†]	80	15.3[†]	55	8.0[†]

[†] Denotes a significantly higher rate than the U.S. rate.

Figure 11

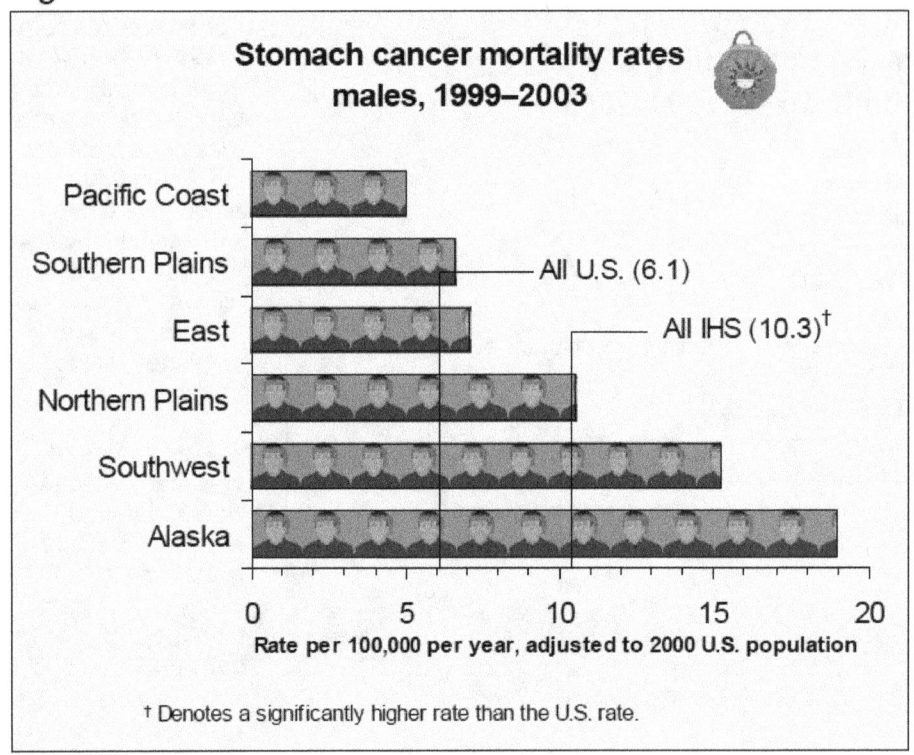

Stomach cancer mortality rates males, 1999–2003

Pacific Coast
Southern Plains — All U.S. (6.1)
East — All IHS (10.3)†
Northern Plains
Southwest
Alaska

Rate per 100,000 per year, adjusted to 2000 U.S. population

† Denotes a significantly higher rate than the U.S. rate.

For males, the 1999–2003 age-adjusted cancer mortality rate for stomach cancer is 10.3/100,000 among the entire IHS service population. This rate is significantly higher than the U.S. all-race combined rate for males.

Regional rates reveal that the Alaska, Southwest, and Northern Plains regions have significantly higher rates than the U.S. rate for males.

Figure 12

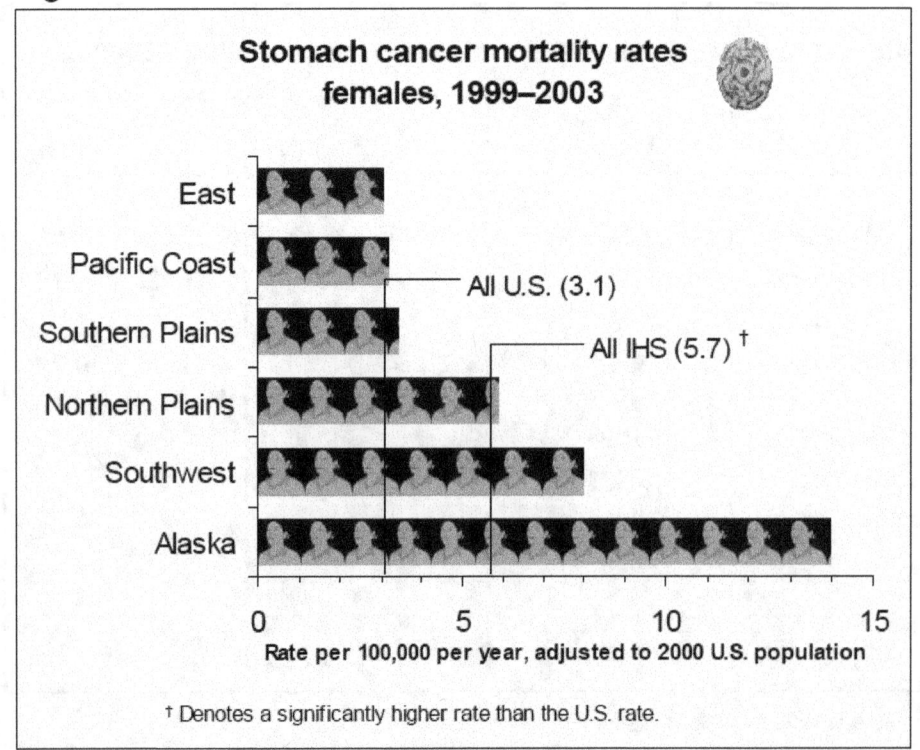

Stomach cancer mortality rates females, 1999–2003

East
Pacific Coast
Southern Plains — All U.S. (3.1)
Northern Plains — All IHS (5.7) †
Southwest
Alaska

Rate per 100,000 per year, adjusted to 2000 U.S. population

† Denotes a significantly higher rate than the U.S. rate.

For females, the 1999–2003 age-adjusted cancer mortality rate for stomach cancer is 5.7/100,000 among the entire IHS service population. This rate is significantly higher than the U.S. all-race combined rate for females.

Regional rates reveal that the Alaska, Southwest, and Northern Plains regions have significantly higher rates than the U.S. rate for females.

Figure 13

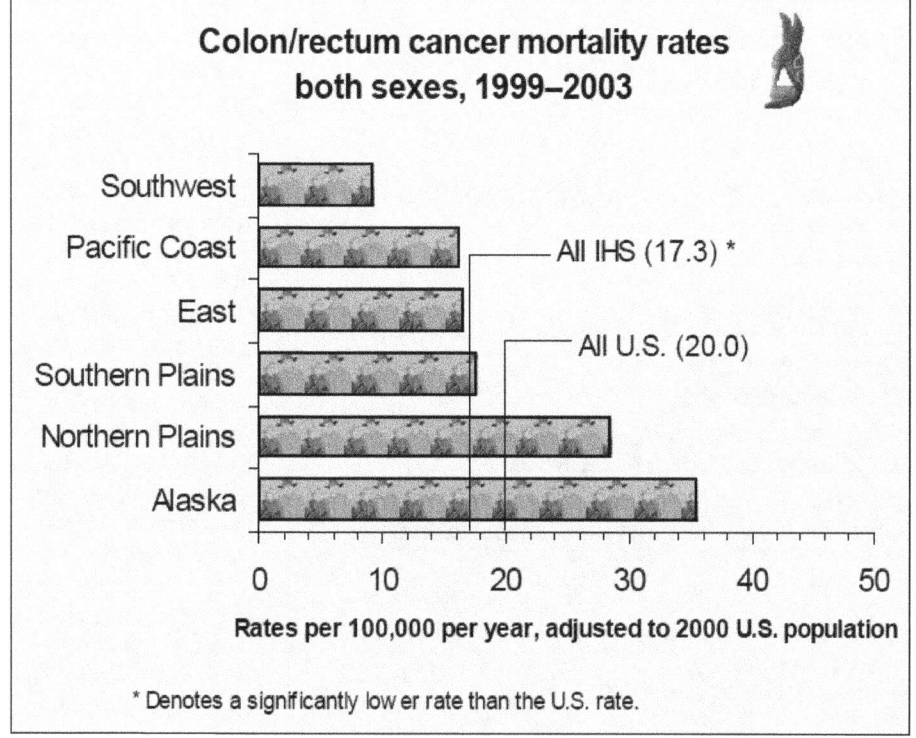

Colon/rectum cancer mortality rates both sexes, 1999–2003

Southwest
Pacific Coast — All IHS (17.3) *
East
Southern Plains — All U.S. (20.0)
Northern Plains
Alaska

0   10   20   30   40   50

Rates per 100,000 per year, adjusted to 2000 U.S. population

* Denotes a significantly lower rate than the U.S. rate.

For both sexes combined, the 1999–2003 age-adjusted cancer mortality rate for colon/rectum cancer is 17.3/100,000 among the entire IHS service population. This rate is significantly lower than the U.S. all-race combined rate for both sexes.

Regional rates reveal that both the Alaska and Northern Plains regions have significantly higher rates than the U.S. rate. The Southwest and Pacific Coast regions have significantly lower rates than the U.S. rate for both sexes.

Table 5

Table 5 lists the total number of deaths caused by colorectal cancer, 1999–2003, as well as mortality rates by IHS region for both sexes combined, males, and females.

Mortality rates are calculated per 100,000/ year and are age-adjusted to the 2000 U.S. population. Rates based on limited numbers of deaths should be interpreted with caution.

Colon/rectum cancer mortality rates and total number of deaths, 1999–2003						
	Both sexes		Males		Females	
	No.	Rate	No.	Rate	No.	Rate
U.S. all races	283,850	20.0	141,487	24.3	142,363	17.0
All IHS regions	753	17.3*	394	20.9*	359	14.8*
Alaska	90	35.5†	47	45.4†	43	30.5†
East	49	16.6	21	13.8*	28	17.9
Northern Plains	159	28.6†	80	37.1†	79	24.4†
Pacific Coast	144	16.4*	81	21.0	63	13.0*
Southern Plains	179	17.8	92	21.5	87	15.1
Southwest	132	9.4*	73	11.4*	59	7.9*

* Denotes a significantly lower rate than the U.S. rate.
† Denotes a significantly higher rate than the U.S. rate.

Figure 14

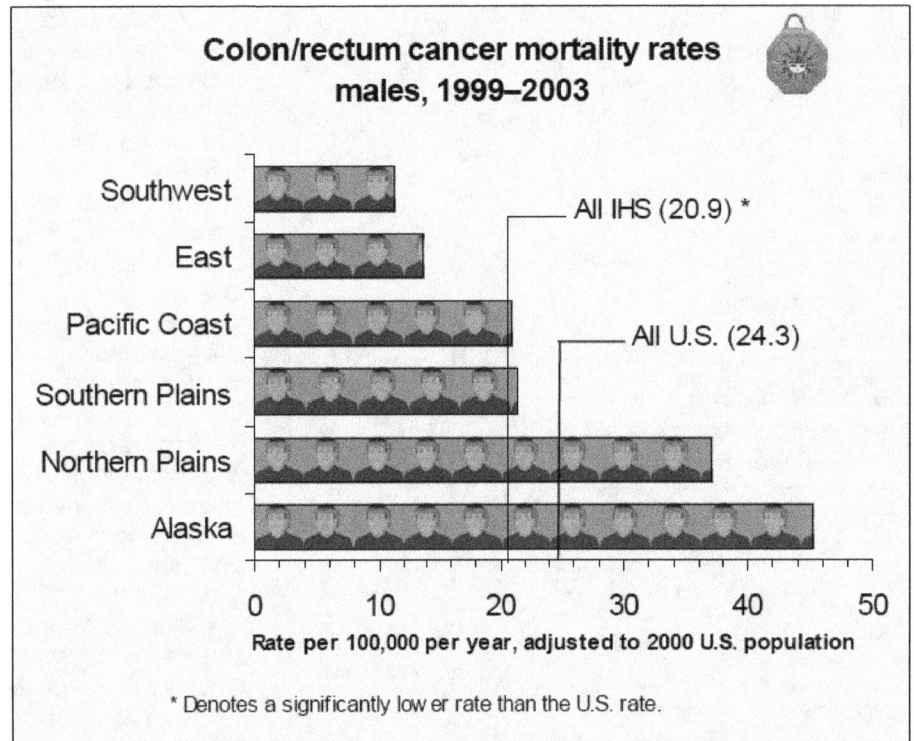

Colon/rectum cancer mortality rates males, 1999–2003

All IHS (20.9) *

All U.S. (24.3)

Rate per 100,000 per year, adjusted to 2000 U.S. population

* Denotes a significantly low er rate than the U.S. rate.

For males, the 1999–2003 age-adjusted cancer mortality rate for colon/rectum cancer is 20.9/100,000 among the entire IHS service population. This rate is significantly lower than the U.S. all-race combined rate for males.

Regional rates reveal that both the Alaska and Northern Plains regions have significantly higher rates than the U.S. rate. The Southwest and East regions have significantly lower rates than the U.S. rate for males.

Figure 15

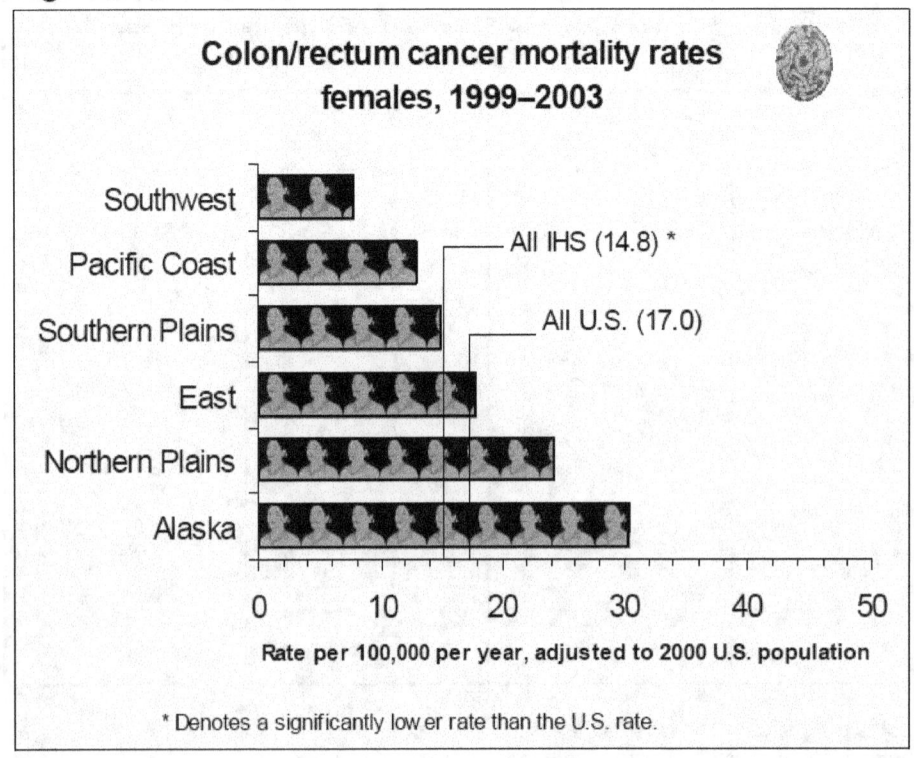

Colon/rectum cancer mortality rates females, 1999–2003

All IHS (14.8) *

All U.S. (17.0)

Rate per 100,000 per year, adjusted to 2000 U.S. population

* Denotes a significantly low er rate than the U.S. rate.

For females, the 1999–2003 age-adjusted cancer mortality rate for colon/rectum cancer is 14.8/100,000 over the entire IHS service population. This rate is significantly lower than the U.S. all-race combined rate for females.

Regional rates reveal that both the Alaska and Northern Plains regions have significantly higher rates than the U.S. rate. The Southwest and Pacific Coast regions have significantly lower rates than the U.S. rate for females.

Figure 16

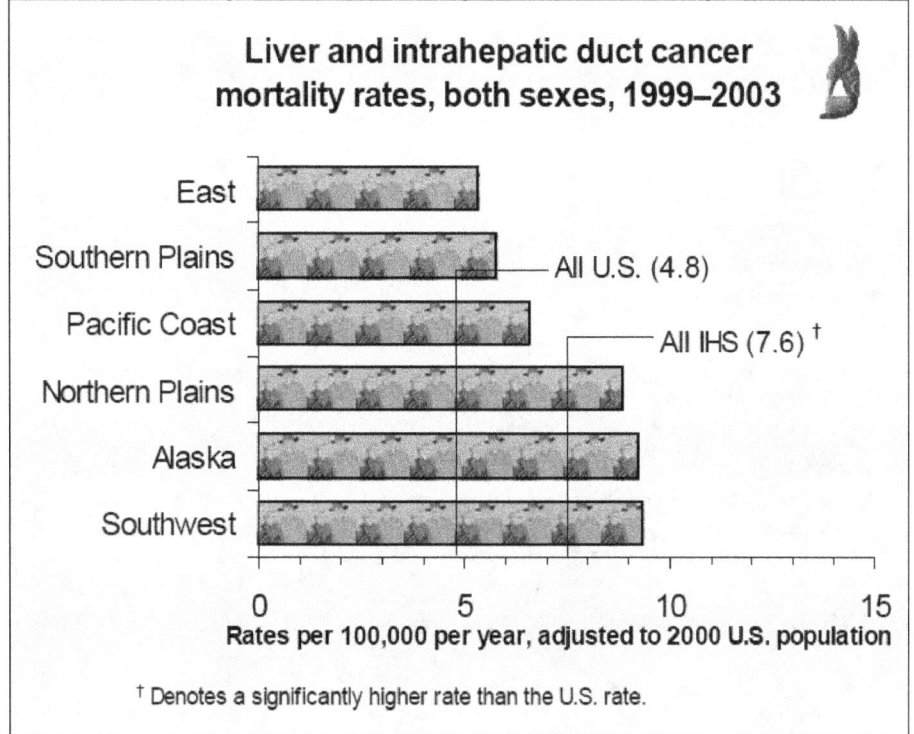

Liver and intrahepatic duct cancer mortality rates, both sexes, 1999–2003

East
Southern Plains — All U.S. (4.8)
Pacific Coast — All IHS (7.6) †
Northern Plains
Alaska
Southwest

0   5   10   15

Rates per 100,000 per year, adjusted to 2000 U.S. population

† Denotes a significantly higher rate than the U.S. rate.

For both sexes combined, the 1999–2003 age-adjusted cancer mortality rate for liver and intrahepatic duct cancer is 7.6/100,000 among the entire IHS service population. This rate is significantly higher than the U.S. all-race combined rate for both sexes.

Regional rates reveal that four regions (Southwest, Alaska, Northern Plains, Pacific Coast) have significantly higher rates than the U.S. rate for both sexes.

Table 6

Table 6 lists the total number of deaths caused by liver and intrahepatic duct cancer, 1999–2003, as well as mortality rates by IHS region for both sexes combined, males, and females.

Mortality rates are calculated per 100,000/year and are age-adjusted to the 2000 U.S. population. Rates based on limited numbers of deaths should be interpreted with caution.

Liver and intrahepatic duct cancer mortality rates and total number of deaths, 1999–2003						
	Both sexes		Males		Females	
	No.	Rate	No.	Rate	No.	Rate
U.S. all races	67,402	4.8	42,841	7.0	24,561	3.0
All IHS regions	346	7.6†	212	10.0†	134	5.6†
Alaska	26	9.3†	11	8.4	15	10.1†
East	17	5.4	11	7.0	6	3.9
Northern Plains	58	8.9†	42	13.6†	16	4.9
Pacific Coast	63	6.6†	32	6.9	31	6.1†
Southern Plains	61	5.8	37	7.7	24	4.2
Southwest	121	9.4†	79	13.4†	42	6.1†

† Denotes a significantly higher rate than the U.S. rate.

Figure 17

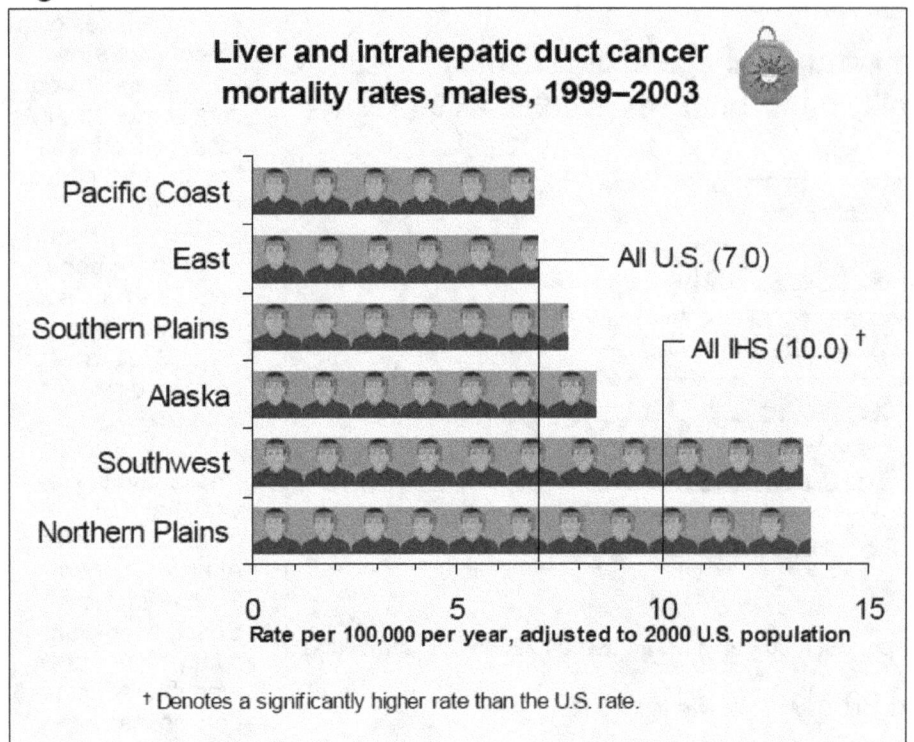

Liver and intrahepatic duct cancer mortality rates, males, 1999–2003

Pacific Coast
East — All U.S. (7.0)
Southern Plains
Alaska — All IHS (10.0) †
Southwest
Northern Plains

0   5   10   15
Rate per 100,000 per year, adjusted to 2000 U.S. population

† Denotes a significantly higher rate than the U.S. rate.

For males, the 1999–2003 age-adjusted cancer mortality rate for liver and intrahepatic duct cancer is 10.0/100,000 among the entire IHS service population. This rate is significantly higher than the U.S. all-race combined rate for males.

Regional rates reveal that both the Northern Plains and Southwest regions have significantly higher rates than the U.S. rate for males.

Figure 18

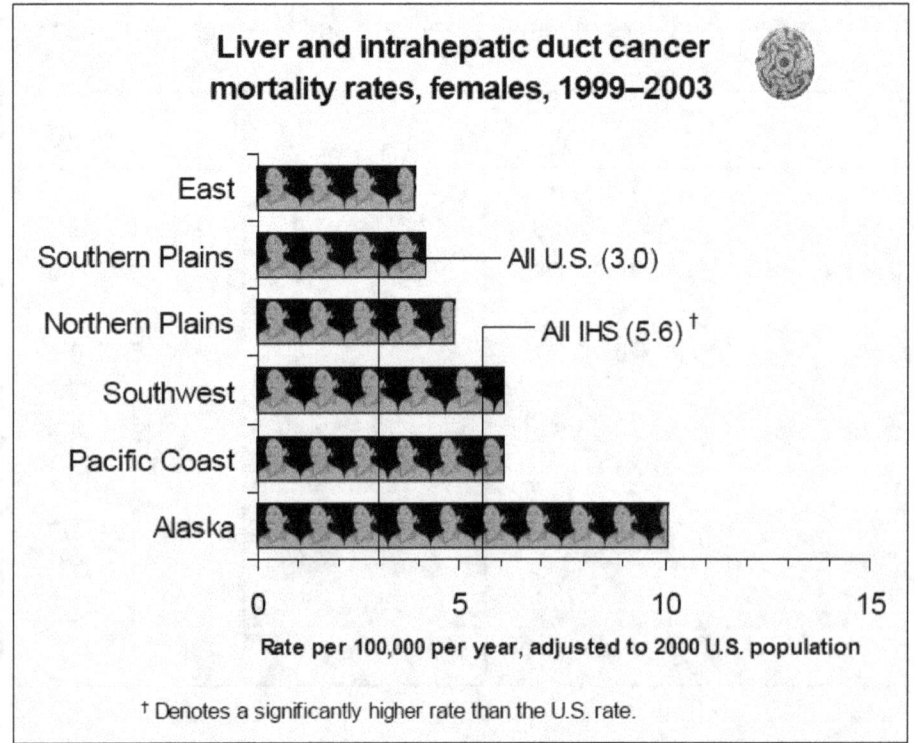

Liver and intrahepatic duct cancer mortality rates, females, 1999–2003

East
Southern Plains — All U.S. (3.0)
Northern Plains — All IHS (5.6) †
Southwest
Pacific Coast
Alaska

0   5   10   15
Rate per 100,000 per year, adjusted to 2000 U.S. population

† Denotes a significantly higher rate than the U.S. rate.

For females, the 1999–2003 age-adjusted cancer mortality rate for colon/rectum cancer is 5.6/100,000 among the entire IHS service population. This rate is significantly higher than the U.S. all-race combined rate for females.

Regional rates reveal that the Alaska, Pacific Coast, and Southwest regions have significantly higher rates than the U.S. rate for females.

Figure 19

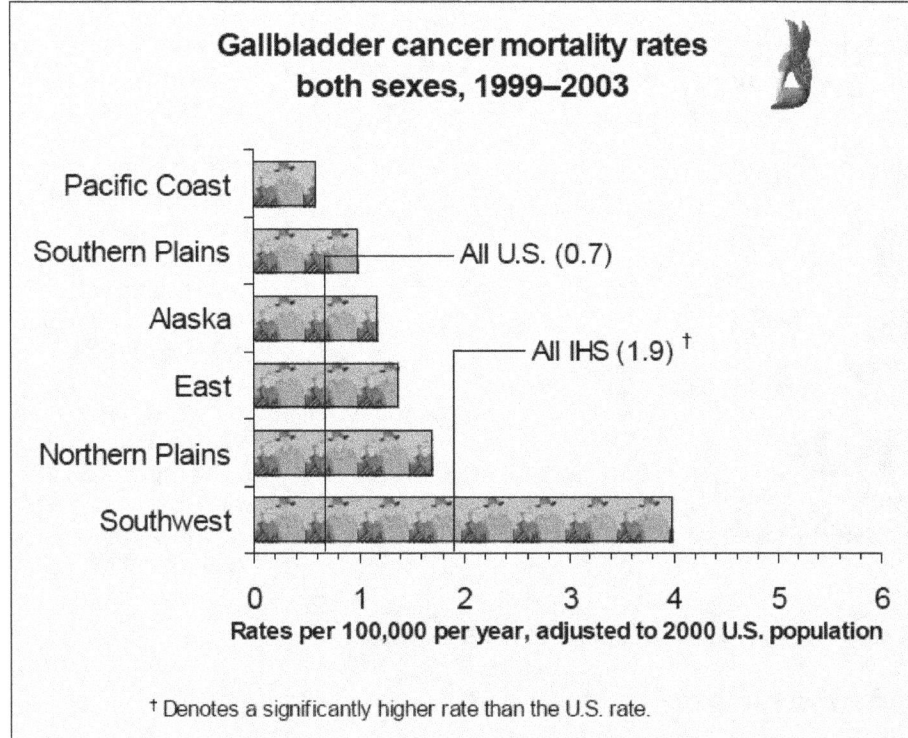

For both sexes combined, the 1999–2003 age-adjusted cancer mortality rate for gallbladder cancer is 1.9/100,000 among the entire IHS service population. This rate is significantly higher than the U.S. all-race combined rate for both sexes.

Regional rates reveal that Southwest and Northern Plains regions have significantly higher rates than the U.S. rate for both sexes.

Table 7

Table 7 lists the total number of deaths caused by gallbladder cancer, 1999–2003, as well as mortality rates by IHS region for both sexes combined, males, and females.

Mortality rates are calculated per 100,000/year and are age-adjusted to the 2000 U.S. population. Rates based on limited numbers of deaths should be interpreted with caution.

	Both sexes		Males		Females	
	No.	Rate	No.	Rate	No.	Rate
U.S. all races	9,801	0.7	2,868	0.5	6,933	0.8
All IHS regions	79	1.9†	19	1.2†	60	2.5†
Alaska	3	1.2	1	0.8	2	1.5
East	3	1.4	1	1.5	2	1.5
Northern Plains	10	1.7†	2	0.7	8	2.4†
Pacific Coast	5	0.6	0	0.0	5	1.0
Southern Plains	9	1.0	3	0.9	6	1.1
Southwest	49	4.0†	12	2.5†	37	5.1†

Gallbladder cancer mortality rates and total number of deaths, 1999–2003

† Denotes a significantly higher rate than the U.S. rate.

27

Figure 20

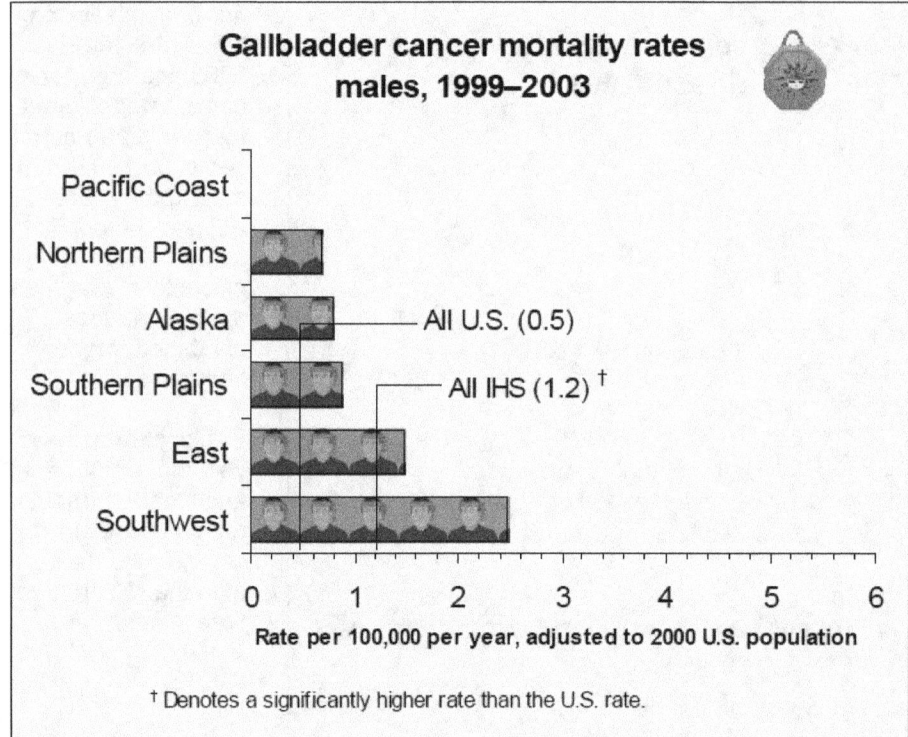

Gallbladder cancer mortality rates males, 1999–2003

Region	
Pacific Coast	
Northern Plains	
Alaska	— All U.S. (0.5)
Southern Plains	— All IHS (1.2) [†]
East	
Southwest	

Rate per 100,000 per year, adjusted to 2000 U.S. population

[†] Denotes a significantly higher rate than the U.S. rate.

For males, the 1999–2003 age-adjusted cancer mortality rate for gallbladder cancer is 1.2/100,000 among the entire IHS service population. This rate is significantly higher than the U.S. all-race combined rate for males.

Regional rates reveal that the Southwest region has a significantly higher rate than the U.S. rate for males.

Figure 21

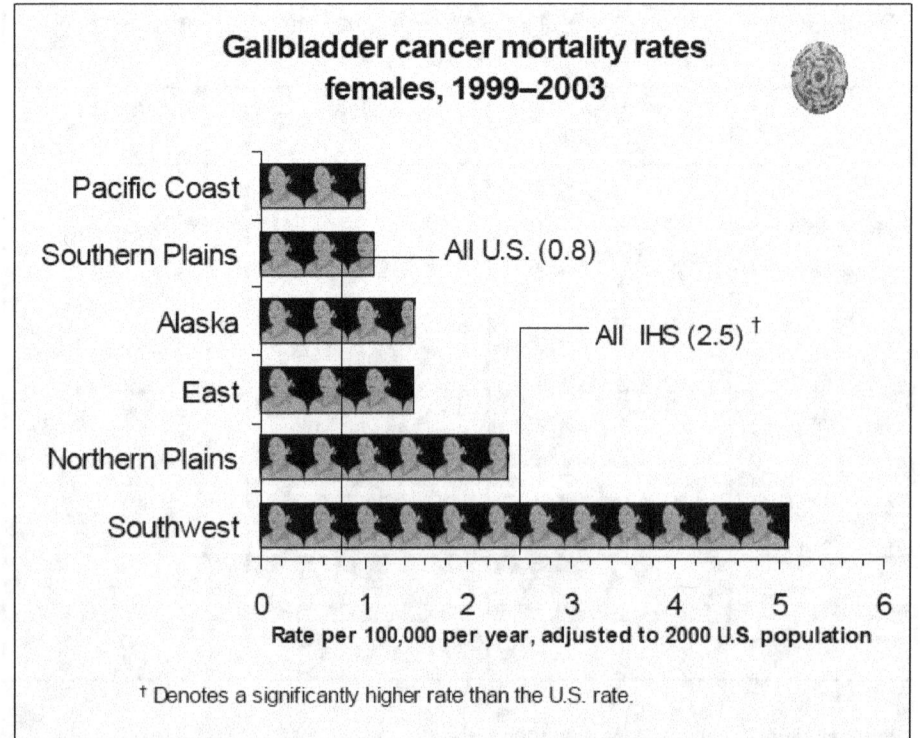

Gallbladder cancer mortality rates females, 1999–2003

Region	
Pacific Coast	
Southern Plains	— All U.S. (0.8)
Alaska	
East	— All IHS (2.5) [†]
Northern Plains	
Southwest	

Rate per 100,000 per year, adjusted to 2000 U.S. population

[†] Denotes a significantly higher rate than the U.S. rate.

For females, the 1999–2003 age-adjusted cancer mortality rate for gallbladder cancer is 2.5/100,000 among the entire IHS service population. This rate is significantly higher than the U.S. all-race combined rate for females.

Regional rates reveal that the Southwest and Northern Plains regions have significantly higher rates than the U.S. rate for females.

28

Figure 22

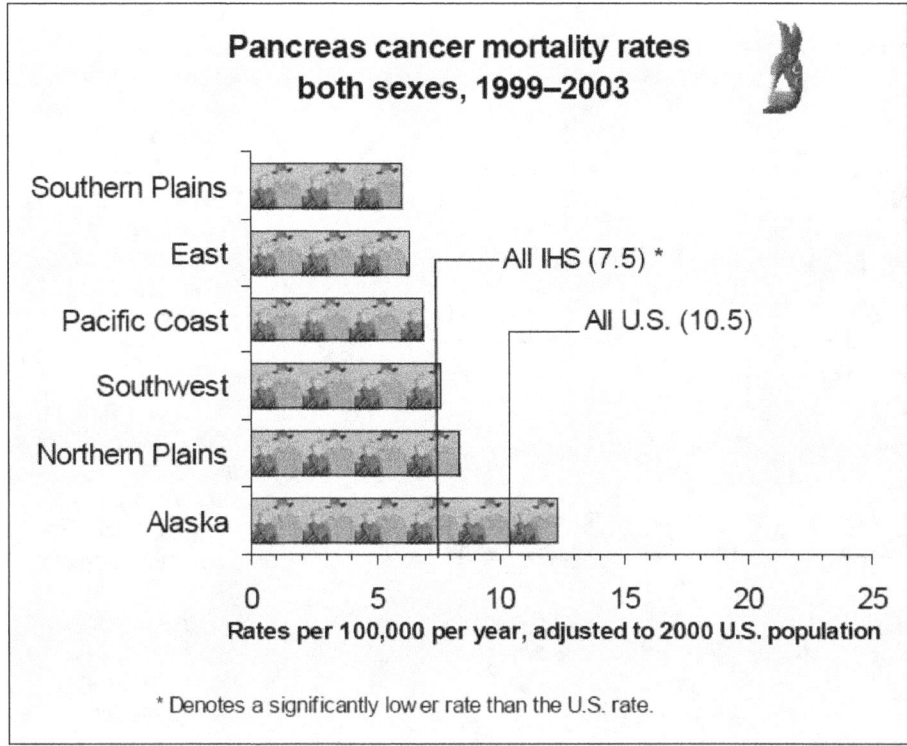

Pancreas cancer mortality rates both sexes, 1999–2003

Southern Plains
East — All IHS (7.5) *
Pacific Coast — All U.S. (10.5)
Southwest
Northern Plains
Alaska

Rates per 100,000 per year, adjusted to 2000 U.S. population

* Denotes a significantly lower rate than the U.S. rate.

For both sexes combined, the 1999–2003 age-adjusted cancer mortality rate for pancreatic cancer is 7.5/100,000 among the entire IHS service population. This rate is significantly lower than the U.S. all-race combined rate for both sexes.

Regional rates reveal that the Southern Plains, East, Pacific Coast, and Southwest regions have significantly lower rates than the U.S. rate for both sexes.

Table 8

Table 8 lists the total number of deaths caused by pancreatic cancer, 1999–2003, as well as mortality rates by IHS region for both sexes combined, males, and females.

Mortality rates are calculated per 100,000/year and are age-adjusted to the 2000 U.S. population. Rates based on limited numbers of deaths should be interpreted with caution.

Pancreas cancer mortality rates and total number of deaths, 1999–2003						
	Both sexes		Males		Females	
	No.	Rate	No.	Rate	No.	Rate
U.S. all races	149,254	10.5	72,815	12.2	76,439	9.2
All IHS regions	329	7.5*	151	7.5*	178	7.4*
Alaska	37	12.4	23	20.0†	14	7.7
East	20	6.4*	10	6.8	10	6.1
Northern Plains	56	8.4	26	7.9*	30	8.5
Pacific Coast	61	7.0*	22	4.8*	39	8.4
Southern Plains	60	6.1*	27	5.7*	33	5.9*
Southwest	95	7.7*	43	7.9*	52	7.5

* Denotes a significantly lower rate than the U.S. rate.
† Denotes a significantly higher rate than the U.S. rate.

Figure 23

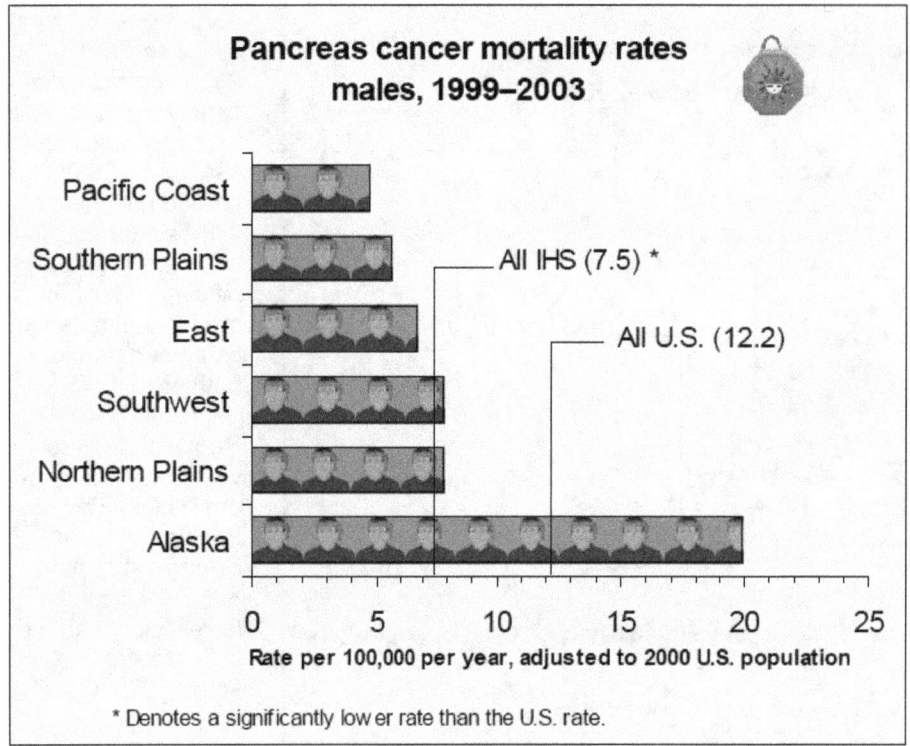

Pancreas cancer mortality rates males, 1999–2003

Pacific Coast
Southern Plains — All IHS (7.5) *
East — All U.S. (12.2)
Southwest
Northern Plains
Alaska

Rate per 100,000 per year, adjusted to 2000 U.S. population

0   5   10   15   20   25

* Denotes a significantly lower rate than the U.S. rate.

For males, the 1999–2003 age-adjusted cancer mortality rate for pancreatic cancer is 7.5/100,000 among the entire IHS service population. This rate is significantly lower than the U.S. all-race combined rate for males.

Regional rates reveal that the Alaska region has a significantly higher rate than the U.S. rate. Four other regions (Pacific Coast, Southern Plains, Southwest, and Northern Plains) have significantly lower rates than the U.S. rate for males.

Figure 24

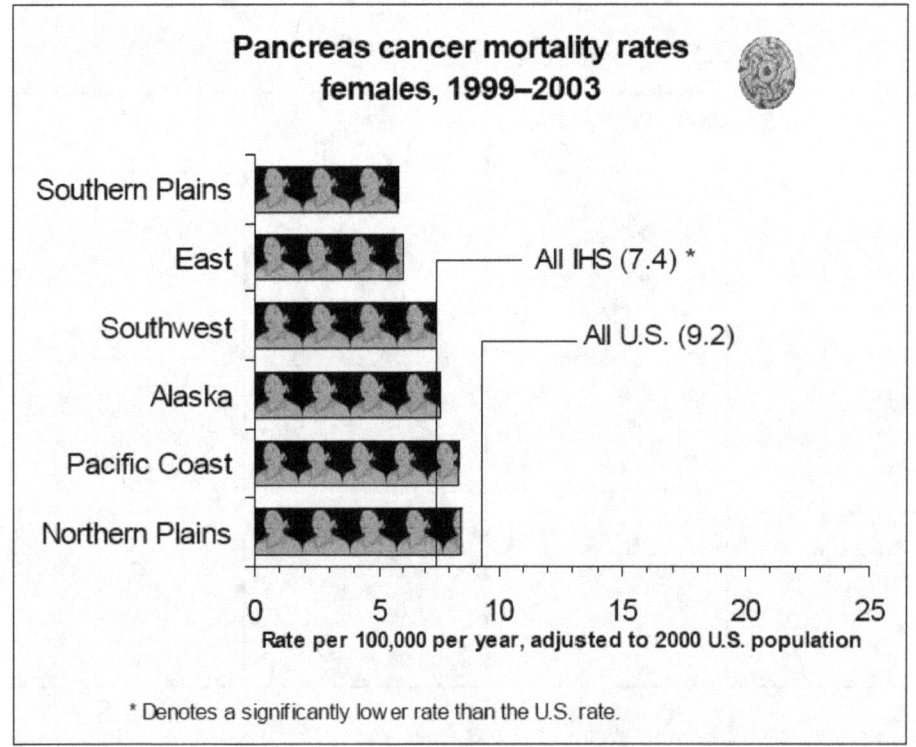

Pancreas cancer mortality rates females, 1999–2003

Southern Plains
East — All IHS (7.4) *
Southwest — All U.S. (9.2)
Alaska
Pacific Coast
Northern Plains

Rate per 100,000 per year, adjusted to 2000 U.S. population

0   5   10   15   20   25

* Denotes a significantly lower rate than the U.S. rate.

For females, the 1999–2003 age-adjusted cancer mortality rate for pancreatic cancer is 7.4/100,000 among the entire IHS service population. This rate is significantly lower than the U.S. all-race combined rate for females.

Regional rates reveal that the Southern Plains region has a significantly lower rate than the U.S. rate for females.

Figure 25

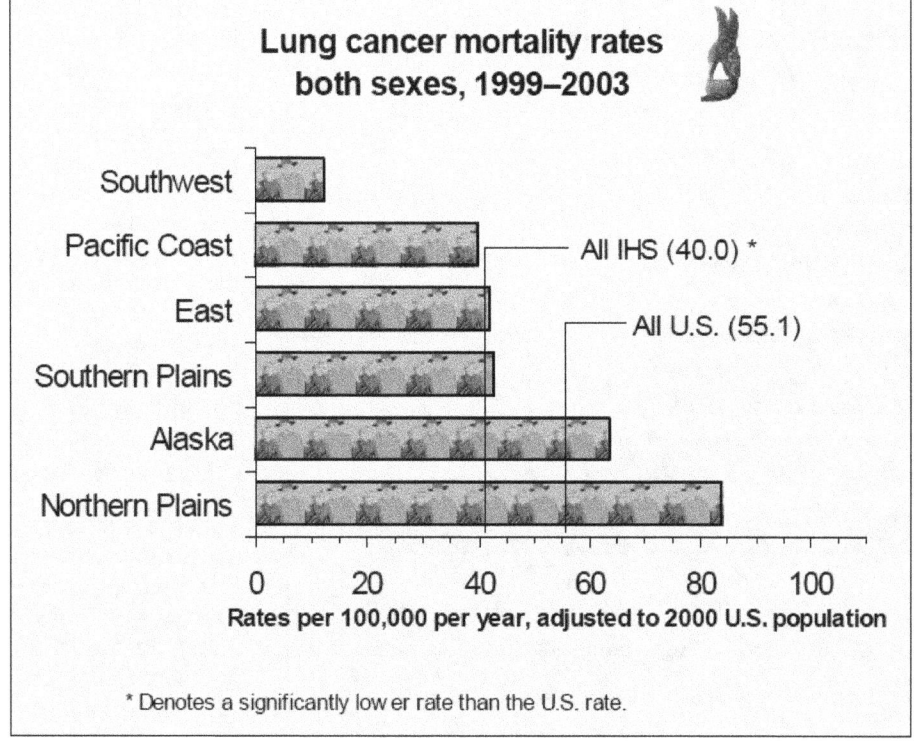

For both sexes combined, the 1999–2003 age-adjusted cancer mortality rate for lung cancer is 40.0/100,000 among the entire IHS service population. This rate is significantly lower than the U.S. all-race combined rate for both sexes.

Regional rates reveal that the Northern Plains region has a significantly higher rate than the U.S. rate for both sexes. Four other regions (Southwest, Pacific Coast, East, and Southern Plains) have significantly lower rates than the U.S. rate for both sexes.

Table 9

Table 9 lists the total number of deaths caused by lung cancer, 1999–2003, as well as mortality rates by IHS region for both sexes combined, males, and females.

Mortality rates are calculated per 100,000/year and are age-adjusted to the 2000 U.S. population. Rates based on limited numbers of deaths should be interpreted with caution.

	Both sexes		Males		Females	
	No.	Rate	No.	Rate	No.	Rate
U.S. all races	779,076	55.1	450,199	74.8	328,877	41.0
All IHS regions	1763	40.0*	951	50.0*	812	32.8*
Alaska	173	63.8	103	82.0	70	49.2
East	123	42.2*	66	51.6*	57	35.5
Northern Plains	505	84.2†	257	100.3†	248	73.2†
Pacific Coast	368	40.3*	189	47.1*	179	35.5
Southern Plains	439	43.0*	243	56.2*	196	33.6*
Southwest	155	12.4*	93	17.9*	62	8.4*

Lung cancer mortality rates and total number of deaths, 1999–2003

* Denotes a significantly lower rate than the U.S. rate.
† Denotes a significantly higher rate than the U.S. rate.

Figure 26

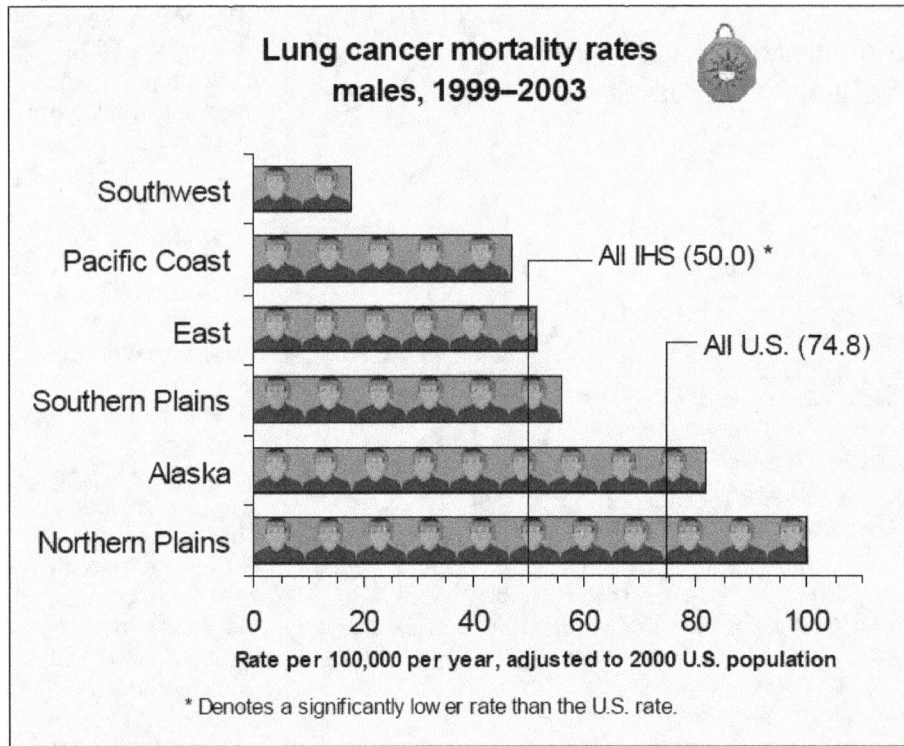

Lung cancer mortality rates males, 1999–2003

- Southwest
- Pacific Coast — All IHS (50.0) *
- East — All U.S. (74.8)
- Southern Plains
- Alaska
- Northern Plains

Rate per 100,000 per year, adjusted to 2000 U.S. population

* Denotes a significantly lower rate than the U.S. rate.

For males, the 1999–2003 age-adjusted cancer mortality rate for lung cancer is 50.0/100,000 among the entire IHS service population. This rate is significantly lower than the U.S. all-race combined rate for males.

Regional rates reveal that the Northern Plains region has a significantly higher rate than the U.S. rate for males. Four other regions (Southwest, Pacific Coast, East, and Southern Plains) have significantly lower rates than the U.S. rate for males.

Figure 27

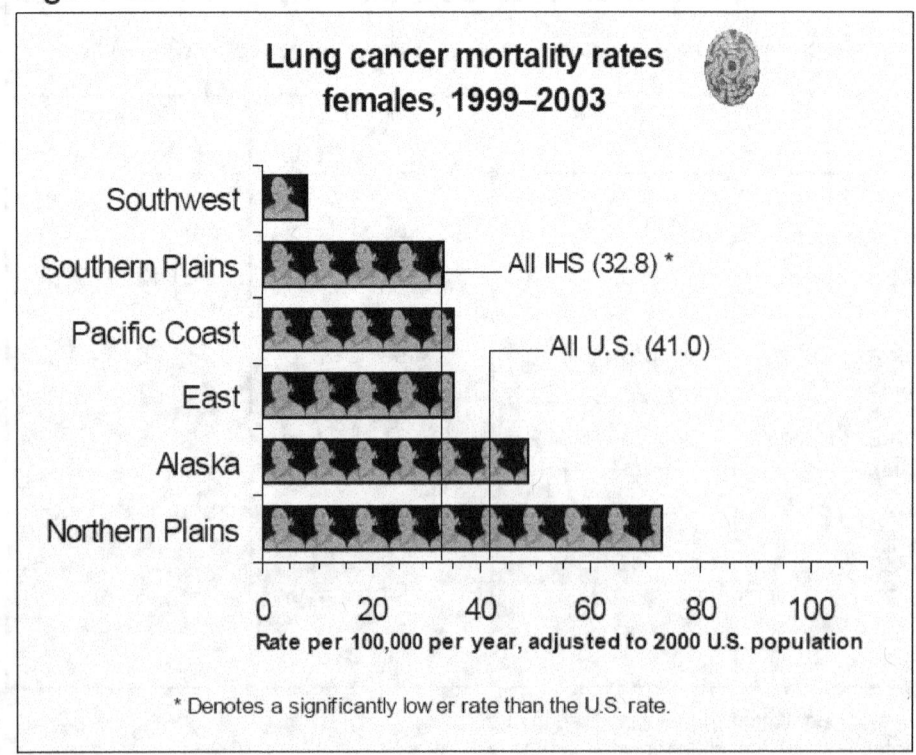

Lung cancer mortality rates females, 1999–2003

- Southwest
- Southern Plains — All IHS (32.8) *
- Pacific Coast — All U.S. (41.0)
- East
- Alaska
- Northern Plains

Rate per 100,000 per year, adjusted to 2000 U.S. population

* Denotes a significantly lower rate than the U.S. rate.

For females, the 1999–2003 age-adjusted cancer mortality rate for lung cancer is 32.8/100,000 among the entire IHS service population. This rate is significantly lower than the U.S. all-race combined rate for females.

Regional rates reveal that the Northern Plains region has a significantly higher rate than the U.S. rate for females. The Southwest and Southern Plains regions have significantly lower rates than the U.S. rate for females.

Figure 28

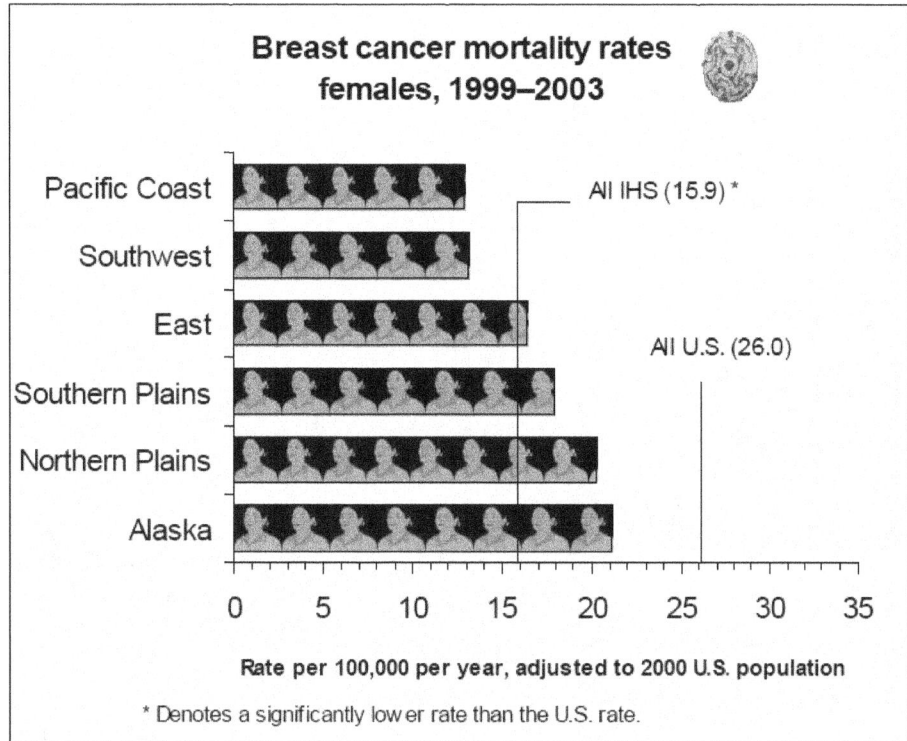

Breast cancer mortality rates females, 1999–2003

Pacific Coast
Southwest
East
Southern Plains
Northern Plains
Alaska

All IHS (15.9) *

All U.S. (26.0)

0 5 10 15 20 25 30 35

Rate per 100,000 per year, adjusted to 2000 U.S. population

* Denotes a significantly lower rate than the U.S. rate.

For females, the 1999–2003 age-adjusted cancer mortality rate for breast cancer is 15.9/100,000 among the entire IHS service population. This rate is significantly lower than the U.S. all-race combined rate for females.

Regional rates reveal that five regions (Pacific Coast, Southwest, East, Southern Plains, and Northern Plains) have significantly lower rates than the U.S. rate for females.

Table 10

Table 10 lists the total number of deaths caused by breast cancer, 1999–2003, as well as mortality rates by IHS region for both sexes combined, males, and females.

Mortality rates are calculated per 100,000/ year and are age-adjusted to the 2000 U.S. population. Rates based on limited numbers of deaths should be interpreted with caution.

Breast cancer mortality rates and total number of deaths, 1999–2003

	Both sexes		Males		Females	
	No.	Rate	No.	Rate	No.	Rate
U.S. all races	209,518	14.8	1,975	0.3	207,543	26.0
All IHS regions	437	9.0*	2	0.1	435	15.9*
Alaska	38	11.4	0	0.0	38	21.2
East	30	9.5*	1	0.7	29	16.5*
Northern Plains	77	11.6	0	0.0	77	20.3*
Pacific Coast	72	7.3*	0	0.0	72	13.0*
Southern Plains	110	10.4*	1	0.4	109	18.0*
Southwest	110	7.4*	0	0.0	110	13.2*

* Denotes a significantly lower rate than the U.S. rate.

Figure 29

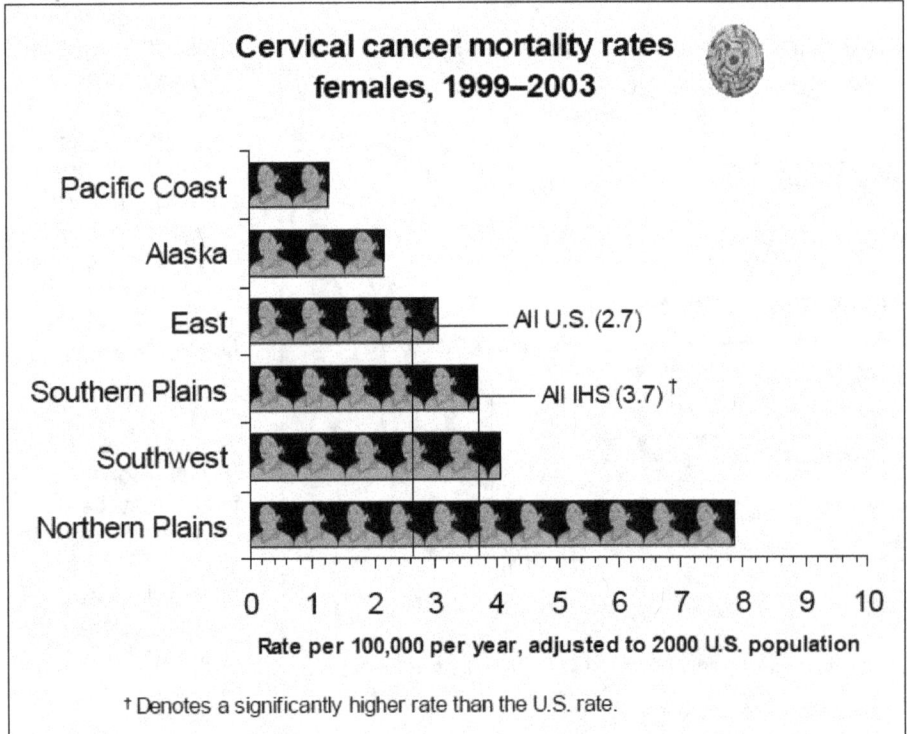

For females, the 1999–2003 age-adjusted cancer mortality rate for cervical cancer is 3.7/100,000 among the entire IHS service population. This rate is significantly higher than the U.S. all-race combined rate for females.

Regional rates reveal that the Northern Plains and Southwest regions have significantly higher rates than the U.S. rate for females.

Table 11

Table 11 lists the total number of deaths caused by cervical cancer, 1999–2003, as well as mortality rates by IHS region for females.

Mortality rates are calculated per 100,000/ year and are age-adjusted to the 2000 U.S. population. Rates based on limited numbers of deaths should be interpreted with caution.

Cervical cancer mortality rates and total number of deaths, 1999–2003		
	Females	
	No.	Rate
U.S. all races	20,367	2.7
All IHS regions	114	3.7[†]
Alaska	4	2.2
East	6	3.1
Northern Plains	35	7.9[†]
Pacific Coast	9	1.3
Southern Plains	25	3.7
Southwest	35	4.1[†]

† Denotes a significantly higher rate than the U.S. rate.

34

Figure 30

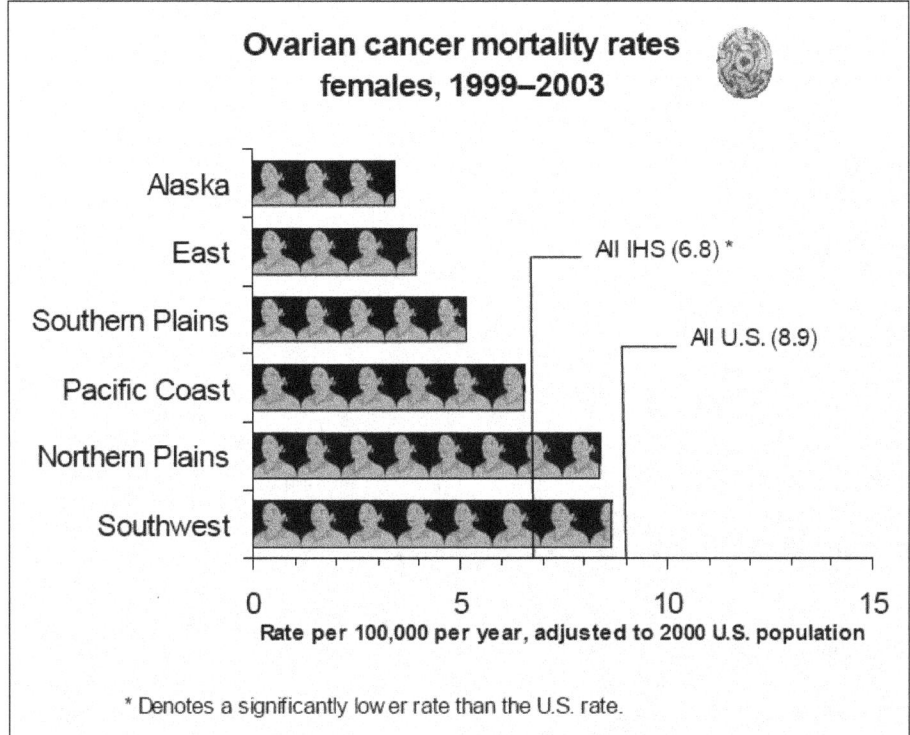

For females, the 1999–2003 age-adjusted cancer mortality rate for ovarian cancer is 6.8/100,000 among the entire IHS service population. This rate is significantly lower than the U.S. all-race combined rate for females.

Regional rates reveal that the Alaska and Southern Plains regions have significantly lower rates than the U.S. rate for females.

Table 12 lists the total number of deaths caused by ovarian cancer, 1999–2003, as well as mortality rates by IHS region for females.

Mortality rates are calculated per 100,000/ year and are age-adjusted to the 2000 U.S. population. Rates based on limited numbers of deaths should be interpreted with caution.

Table 12

Ovarian cancer mortality rates and total number of deaths, 1999–2003		
	Females	
	No.	Rate
U.S. all races	71,440	8.9
All IHS regions	177	6.8*
Alaska	7	3.5*
East	6	4.0
Northern Plains	30	8.4
Pacific Coast	37	6.6
Southern Plains	29	5.2*
Southwest	68	8.7

* Denotes a significantly lower rate than the U.S. rate.

Figure 31

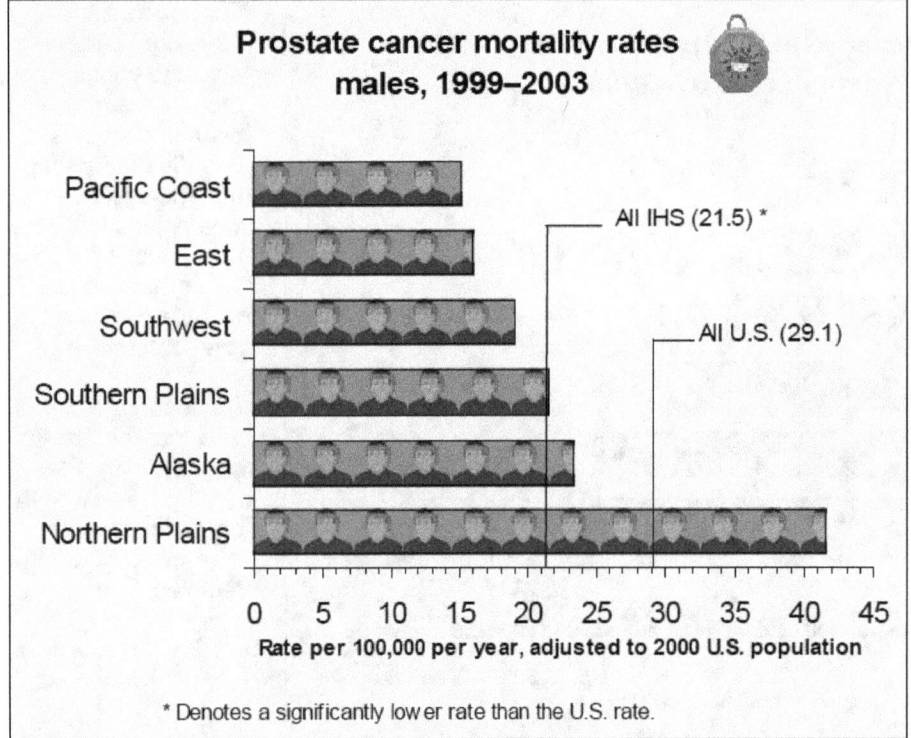

Prostate cancer mortality rates males, 1999–2003

Pacific Coast

East

Southwest

Southern Plains

Alaska

Northern Plains

All IHS (21.5) *

All U.S. (29.1)

0 5 10 15 20 25 30 35 40 45

Rate per 100,000 per year, adjusted to 2000 U.S. population

* Denotes a significantly lower rate than the U.S. rate.

For males, the 1999–2003 age-adjusted cancer mortality rate for prostate cancer is 21.5/100,000 among the entire IHS service population. This rate is significantly lower than the U.S. all-race combined rate for males.

Regional rates reveal that the Northern Plains region has a significantly higher rate than the U.S. rate for males. Four regions (Pacific Coast, East, Southwest, and Southern Plains) have significantly lower rates than the U.S. rate for males.

Table 13

Table 13 lists the total number of deaths caused by prostate cancer, 1999–2003, as well as mortality rates by IHS region for males.

Mortality rates are calculated per 100,000/year and are age-adjusted to the 2000 U.S. population. Rates based on limited numbers of deaths should be interpreted with caution.

Prostate cancer mortality rates and total number of deaths, 1999–2003		
	Males	
	No.	Rate
U.S. all races	153,525	29.1
All IHS regions	293	21.5*
Alaska	14	23.5
East	15	16.1*
Northern Plains	69	41.6†
Pacific Coast	44	15.3*
Southern Plains	69	21.7*
Southwest	82	19.2*

* Denotes a significantly lower rate than the U.S. rate.
† Denotes a significantly higher rate than the U.S. rate.

Figure 32

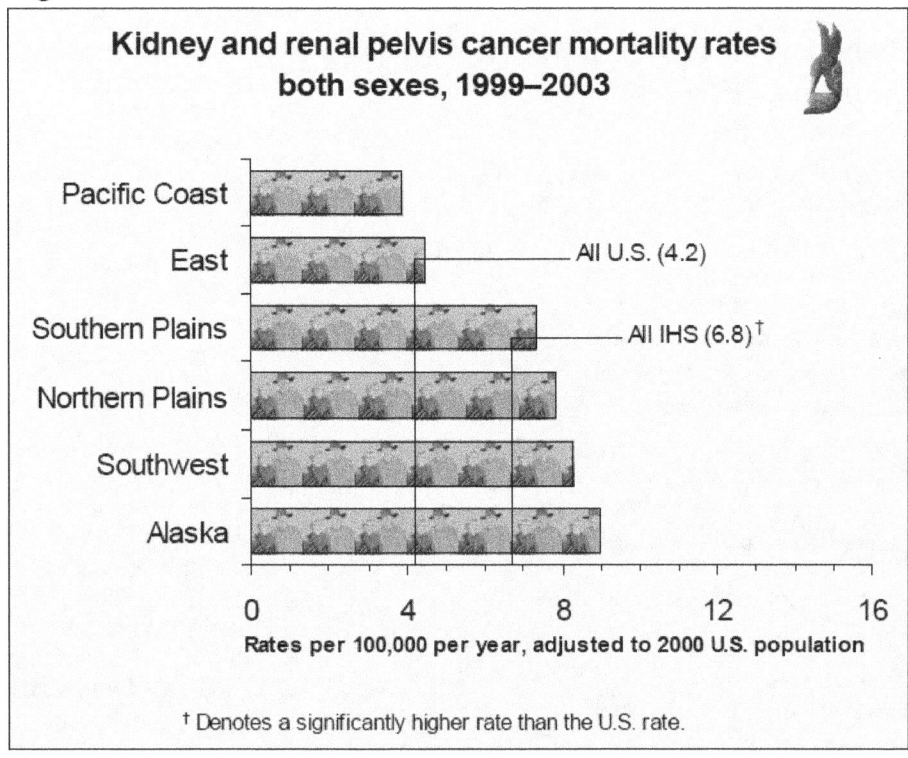

For both sexes combined, the 1999–2003 age-adjusted cancer mortality rate for kidney and renal pelvis cancer is 6.8/100,000 among the entire IHS service population. This rate is significantly higher than the U.S. all-race combined rate for both sexes.

Regional rates reveal that four regions (Alaska, Southwest, Northern Plains, and Southern Plains) have significantly higher rates than the U.S. rate for both sexes.

Table 14

Table 14 lists the total number of deaths caused by kidney and renal pelvis cancer, 1999–2003, as well as mortality rates by IHS region for both sexes combined, males, and females.

Mortality rates are calculated per 100,000/ year and are age-adjusted to the 2000 U.S. population. Rates based on limited numbers of deaths should be interpreted with caution.

Kidney and renal pelvis cancer mortality rates and total number of deaths 1999–2003						
	Both sexes		Males		Females	
	No.	Rate	No.	Rate	No.	Rate
U.S. all races	59,381	4.2	36,894	6.1	22,487	2.8
All IHS regions	320	6.8[†]	202	9.7[†]	118	4.5[†]
Alaska	23	9.0[†]	17	14.9[†]	6	4.3
East	13	4.5	7	5.4	6	3.7
Northern Plains	55	7.9[†]	36	11.3[†]	19	4.9[†]
Pacific Coast	35	3.9	21	5.5	14	2.7
Southern Plains	82	7.4[†]	55	10.8[†]	27	4.4[†]
Southwest	112	8.3[†]	66	11.1[†]	46	6.1[†]

[†] Denotes a significantly higher rate than the U.S. rate.

Figure 33

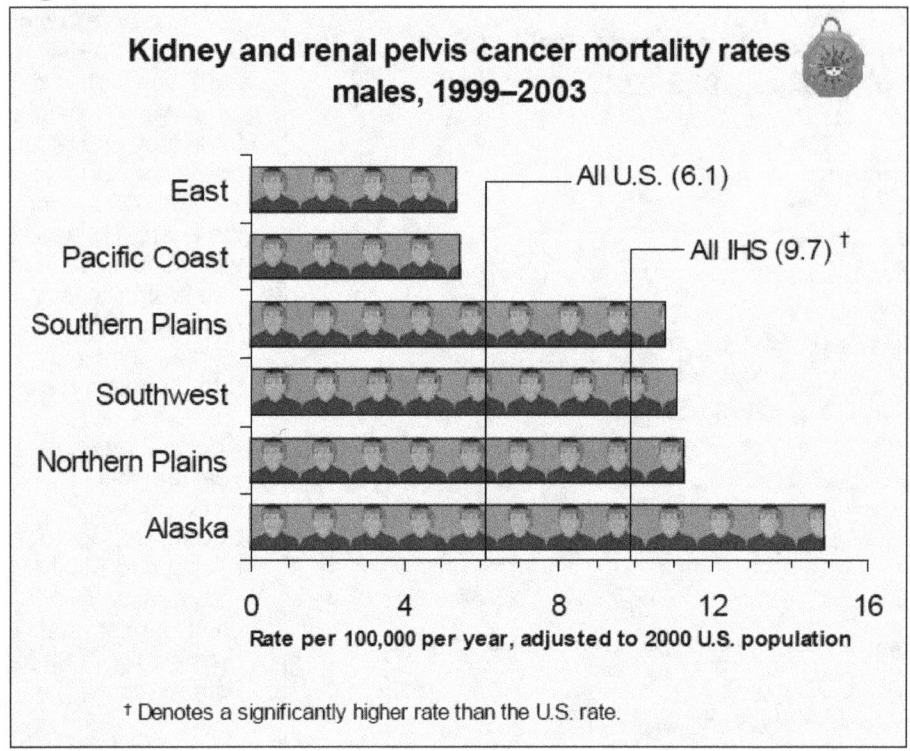

For males, the 1999–2003 age-adjusted cancer mortality rate for kidney and renal pelvis cancer is 9.7/100,000 among the entire IHS service population. This rate is significantly higher than the U.S. all-race combined rate for males.

Regional rates reveal that four regions (Alaska, Northern Plains, Southwest, and Southern Plains) have significantly higher rates than the U.S. rate for males.

Figure 34

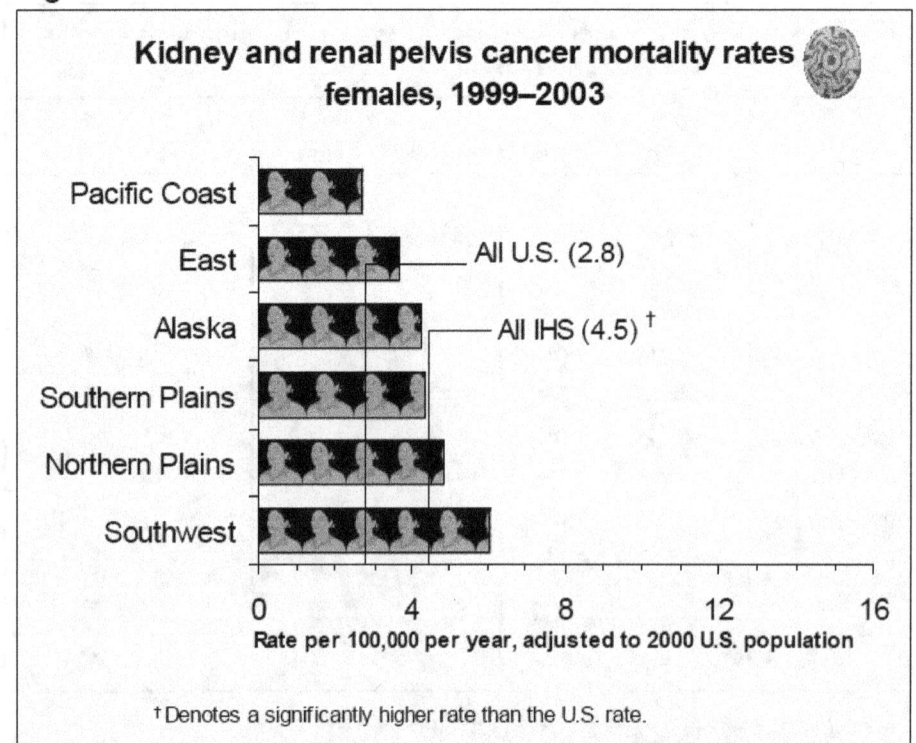

For females, the 1999–2003 age-adjusted cancer mortality rate for kidney and renal pelvis cancer is 4.5/100,000 among the entire IHS service population. This rate is significantly higher than the U.S. all-race combined rate for females.

Regional rates reveal that three regions (Southwest, Northern Plains, and Southern Plains) have significantly higher rates than the U.S. rate for females.

Figure 35

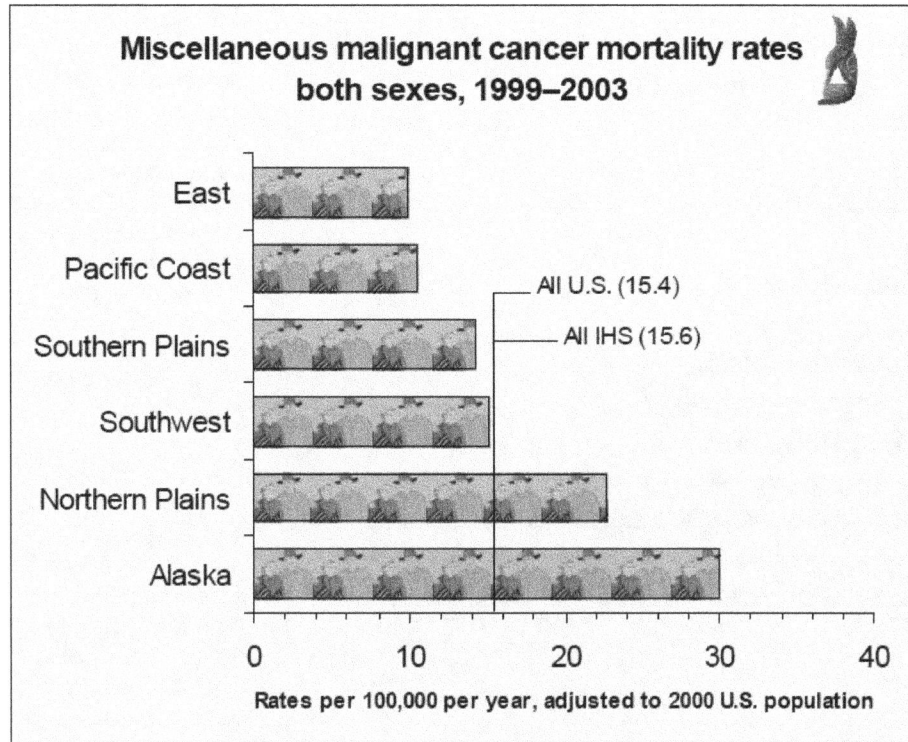

Miscellaneous malignant cancer mortality rates both sexes, 1999–2003

East
Pacific Coast
Southern Plains
Southwest
Northern Plains
Alaska

All U.S. (15.4)
All IHS (15.6)

0   10   20   30   40

Rates per 100,000 per year, adjusted to 2000 U.S. population

For both sexes combined, the 1999–2003 age-adjusted cancer mortality rate for miscellaneous malignant cancer is 15.6/100,000 among the entire IHS service population. This rate is not significantly different than the U.S. all-race combined rate for both sexes.

Regional rates reveal that the Alaska and Northern Plains regions have significantly higher rates than the U.S. rate for both sexes. The East and Pacific Coast regions have significantly lower rates than the U.S. rate for both sexes.

Table 15

Table 15 lists the total number of deaths caused by miscellaneous malignant cancer, 1999–2003, as well as mortality rates by IHS region for both sexes combined, males, and females.

Mortality rates are calculated per 100,000/ year and are age-adjusted to the 2000 U.S. population. Rates based on limited numbers of deaths should be interpreted with caution.

Miscellaneous malignant cancer mortality rates and total number of deaths 1999–2003						
	Both sexes		Males		Females	
	No.	Rate	No.	Rate	No.	Rate
U.S. all races	218,485	15.4	114,094	19.4	104,391	12.6
All IHS regions	674	15.6	347	18.1	327	13.6
Alaska	79	30.1[†]	45	38.0[†]	34	23.6[†]
East	27	10.0[*]	10	8.2[*]	17	11.3
Northern Plains	134	22.8[†]	71	27.0[†]	63	19.6[†]
Pacific Coast	94	10.7[*]	49	12.4[*]	45	9.3
Southern Plains	146	14.4	81	19.1	65	11.3
Southwest	194	15.2	91	16.0	103	14.3

* Denotes a significantly lower rate than the U.S. rate.
† Denotes a significantly higher rate than the U.S. rate.

39

Figure 36

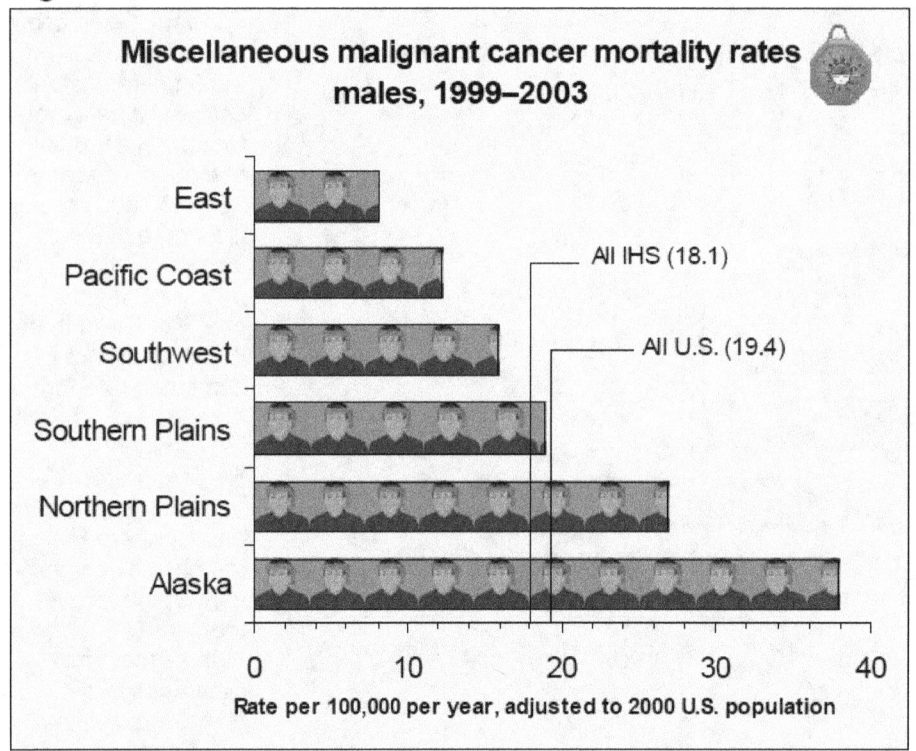

Miscellaneous malignant cancer mortality rates males, 1999–2003

- East
- Pacific Coast — All IHS (18.1)
- Southwest — All U.S. (19.4)
- Southern Plains
- Northern Plains
- Alaska

0   10   20   30   40

Rate per 100,000 per year, adjusted to 2000 U.S. population

For males, the 1999–2003 age-adjusted cancer mortality rate for miscellaneous malignant cancer is 18.1/100,000 among the entire IHS service population. This rate is not significantly different than the U.S. all-race combined rate for males.

Regional rates reveal that the Alaska and Northern Plains regions have significantly higher rates than the U.S. rate for males. The East and Pacific Coast regions have significantly lower rates than the U.S. rate for males.

Figure 37

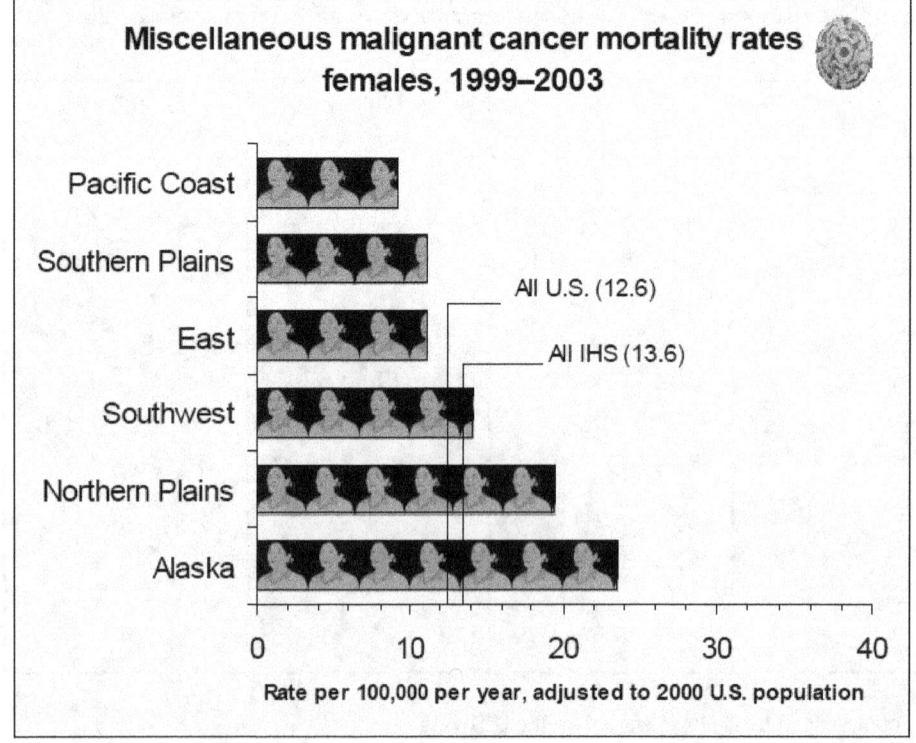

Miscellaneous malignant cancer mortality rates females, 1999–2003

- Pacific Coast
- Southern Plains
- East — All U.S. (12.6)
- Southwest — All IHS (13.6)
- Northern Plains
- Alaska

0   10   20   30   40

Rate per 100,000 per year, adjusted to 2000 U.S. population

For females, the 1999–2003 age-adjusted cancer mortality rate for miscellaneous malignant cancer is 13.6/100,000 among the entire IHS service population. This rate is not significantly different than the U.S. all-race combined rate for females.

Regional rates reveal that the Alaska and Northern Plains regions have significantly higher rates than the U.S. rate for females.

Table 16. Five leading causes of cancer mortality by average annual age-adjusted rates,* 1999–2003, by IHS geographic region and sex, compared with U.S. All races population.

Region	Both sexes		Males		Females	
U.S. All races	Lung	55.1	Lung	74.8	Lung	41.0
	Colon/rectum	20.0	Prostate	29.1	Breast	26.0
	Miscellaneous	15.4	Colon/rectum	24.3	Colon/rectum	17.0
	Breast	14.8	Miscellaneous	19.4	Miscellaneous	12.6
	Prostate	10.9	Pancreas	12.2	Pancreas	9.2
All IHS regions	Lung	40.0	Lung	50.0	Lung	32.8
	Colon/rectum	17.3	Prostate	21.5	Breast	15.9
	Miscellaneous	15.6	Colon/rectum	20.9	Colon/rectum	14.8
	Breast	9.0	Miscellaneous	18.1	Miscellaneous	13.6
	Prostate	8.3	Stomach	10.3	Pancreas	7.4
Alaska	Lung	63.8	Lung	82.0	Lung	49.2
	Colon/rectum	35.5	Colon/rectum	45.4	Colon/rectum	30.5
	Miscellaneous	30.1	Miscellaneous	38.0	Miscellaneous	23.6
	Stomach	15.7	Prostate	23.5	Breast	21.2
	Pancreas	12.4	Pancreas	20.0	Stomach	14.0
East	Lung	42.2	Lung	51.6	Lung	35.5
	Colon/rectum	16.6	Prostate	16.1	Colon/rectum	17.9
	Miscellaneous	10.0	Colon/rectum	13.8	Breast	16.5
	Breast	9.5	Miscellaneous	8.2	Miscellaneous	11.3
	Pancreas	6.4	Leukemia	7.7	Pancreas	6.1
Northern Plains	Lung	84.2	Lung	100.3	Lung	73.2
	Colon/rectum	28.6	Prostate	41.6	Colon/rectum	24.4
	Miscellaneous	22.8	Colon/rectum	37.1	Breast	20.3
	Prostate	15.3	Miscellaneous	27.0	Miscellaneous	19.6
	Breast	11.6	Liver	13.6	Pancreas	8.5
Pacific Coast	Lung	40.3	Lung	47.1	Lung	35.5
	Colon/rectum	16.4	Colon/rectum	21.1	Colon/rectum	13.0
	Miscellaneous	10.7	Prostate	15.3	Breast	13.0
	Breast	7.3	Miscellaneous	12.4	Miscellaneous	9.3
	Pancreas	7.0	Leukemia	7.4	Pancreas	8.4
Southern Plains	Lung	43.0	Lung	56.2	Lung	33.6
	Colon/rectum	17.8	Prostate	21.7	Breast	18.0
	Miscellaneous	14.4	Colon/rectum	21.5	Colon/rectum	15.1
	Breast	10.4	Miscellaneous	19.1	Miscellaneous	11.3
	Prostate	7.9	Kidney	10.8	Pancreas	5.9
Southwest	Miscellaneous	15.2	Prostate	19.2	Miscellaneous	14.3
	Lung	12.4	Lung	17.9	Breast	13.2
	Stomach	11.0	Miscellaneous	16.0	Ovary	8.7
	Colon/rectum	9.4	Stomach	15.3	Lung	8.4
	Liver	9.4	Liver	13.4	Stomach	8.0

*All rates are per 100,000 population/year, adjusted to the 2000 U.S. standard population.

41